When Caring Trumps Curing

The Vital Role of Palliative & Hospice Care

Bradley C. Buckhout, M.D.

When Caring Trumps Curing

Copyright @Bradley C. Buckhout, M.D. 2018
All rights reserved.

Bradley C. Buckhout, M.D.

This book is dedicated to my wife, Karen. She has been my constant, my inspiration, my first mate, the love of my life and the one that I have entrusted to be my surrogate decision maker at some distant future time, if my faculties have abandoned me. I would also like to recognize America's veterans for their service, sacrifice and dignity in the face of unfathomable challenges. My years of caring for them have been an honor and their strength and resolve have been the inspiration for this work.

Table of Contents

Chapter 1 Harry's Heart & Che Che to the End 1

Chapter 2 Medical Advances 12

Chapter 3 Advanced Care Planning 20

Chapter 4 The Price of Freedom is Visible Here 30

Part 2

Chapter 5 Emil 33

Chapter 6 Lynn 48

Chapter 7 Tami 63

Chapter 8 Opiates and Pain Control 77

Chapter 9 Jeff 84

Chapter 10 Don 105

Chapter 11 The Story of Juan and Jack 118

Chapter 12 Mr. Gary 123

Chapter 13 Billie 127

Chapter 14 Gratitude, Forgiveness, Apology, Love 145

Chapter 15 Pastor Jefferson and Brother Will 150

Bradley C. Buckhout, M.D.

Appendix A	Life Sustaining Treatment Decision Initiative	168
Appendix B	POLST	171
Appendix C	Resources	179
Notes		181

When Caring Trumps Curing

Bradley C. Buckhout, M.D.

A ship at my side spreads her white sails to the morning breeze
and starts for the blue ocean. She is an object of beauty and strength.
I stand and watch her until at length she hangs like a speck of white cloud
just where the sea and sky come to mingle with each other.

Then someone at my side says: There, she is gone!

Gone where?

Gone from my sight. That is all.

She is just as large in mast and hull and spar
as she was when she left my side and she is just as able to bear
her load of living freight to her destined port.

Her diminished size is in me, not in her.
And just at the moment when someone at my side says:
There, she is gone!
There are other eyes watching her coming,
and other voices ready to take up the glad shout:
Here she comes!

And that is dying.

Author: Henry Van Dyke

Bradley C. Buckhout, M.D.

Chapter 1
Harry's Heart & Che-Che to the End

Harry stares, unseeing, at the white pocked ceiling tiles. The strangers surrounding him seem no longer interested as they remove their purple nitrile gloves and begin to file from the suddenly silent room. Only twenty minutes ago there was a swarm of chaotic action here that was heralded by the calm but authoritative overhead page, "Code Blue...Code Blue...ICU room 6. I repeat Code Blue...ICU room 6."

It seems that Harry's heart, which had served him well for the first 83 years they had shared, had finally lost its will to go on. Three years ago the first portion of this vital muscle was stricken by a plaque that finally occluded a diagonal branch of the left main coronary artery. Harry had recovered with some effort, changed his diet, began to exercise...did the things his cardiologist said would help.

The monitor nurse, alerted by the warbling tone from the bank of displays spotted the tracing from room 6 and recognized ventricular fibrillation, a fatal arrhythmia if not corrected immediately. The bedside nurse rushed to him and found Harry pale, gasping for air and unresponsive. He struck the large crimson Code button near the head of the bed, released the plug on the air mattress, lowered the bed and began CPR.

After the first heart attack Harry was a little more fatigued than normal and his afternoon nap tended to stretch to an hour. He and Vivian were still able to travel, something they very much enjoyed. But he noticed when in Denver visiting their son, shortness of breath was a result of almost any activity. His second episode, seven months after the first, caused the death of another chunk of left ventricle and this time the placement of a coronary artery stent. The cardiologist added more medications to protect this stent. Pill count now sixteen daily…which he usually remembered to take.

With the first downward thrust on the sternum, the nurse, a 230 pound Air Force veteran, heard and felt the snapping of brittle rib cartilages and bone giving way under the pressure needed to compress the heart against the spine. Cardiopulmonary resuscitation was officially introduced in 1969 for witnessed cardiac arrests, ideally in otherwise healthy 50 year olds. It was not intended to be used to reanimate chronically ill, frail geriatric members of the community. However, CPR now is the automatic response of medical personnel and first responders unless you have specified otherwise.

Eighteen months ago a devastating series of hospitalizations began. With each event Harry lost a little more…The pattern became painfully repetitive. Vivian would awake at night to find Harry sitting on the side of the bed, unable to breathe and too weak to walk. The paramedics would come after the 9-1-1 call and the ambulance would transport him, lights flashing, to the ER. The physician on duty would call his cardiologist and he would be readmitted, again.

The code team, led by a senior resident trailing a gaggle of eager, frightened, inexperienced interns and medical students rushes into the room. The resident, inspecting the rhythm strip, asks the nurse for a brief summary of what has happened to Harry as he pulls the defibrillator to the bedside and switches it on. The respiratory therapist and pulmonary resident at the head of the bed tilt Harry's head back and force his jaw open to thrust the

Bradley C. Buckhout, M.D.

laryngoscope blade along the top of his tongue to the back of his throat so that his vocal cords are visible. Once in sight, the plastic endotracheal tube is slipped between the cords and then attached to an ambu bag so that the therapist can begin rhythmically squeezing this bellows to force air into his inanimate lungs.

A recent study published in the American Journal of Geriatrics (1) reviewed the rather dismal outcomes of emergency intubations followed by ventilator support of the aging population. They examined 35,000 patients older than 65 years of age, who presented to emergency rooms in dire straights from a variety of conditions, who ended up needing this intervention. What they discovered was 33% of these older patients died in the hospital and only 24% of the survivors were able to discharge home. So, if one of your recurrent nightmares is that you have become impaired enough that you can no longer care for yourself and will spend the remainder of your days in a nursing home, perhaps you should consider whether you would want to be intubated during your "golden years". Further evaluation of the data shows that, not surprisingly, older patients fare the worst. In the 65-74 age group, 29% died in the hospital and 31% were able to go home. Contrast this with those over 90; 50% of whom died and 14% were well enough to return to their family.

The chest x-rays, repeat angiograms, echocardiograms, lab work, EKGs, physical therapy and occupational therapy became a routine of each hospital admission to which he never adjusted. Medications were added, adjusted or replaced but the pill count continued to increase…twenty-three daily. Even after all of the aggressive care, Harry was too weak to return home directly from the hospital after his admission a month ago. He was admitted to a skilled nursing facility (a nursing home to most people) to receive more physical and occupational therapy. The intention was for Harry to regain enough strength and stamina to be able to return to Vivian and his home where they had lived mostly happily for the last 51 years.

The chief resident applies the defibrillator conductive pads and then the paddles to Harry's bared chest and observes the persistence of the soon to be fatal arrhythmia. "Clear" he calls out and everyone steps back from the bed not wanting to experience the jolt of electricity that will soon cause Harry to involuntarily spasm. The resident triggers the paddles and Harry's body jerks convulsively. The EKG tracing continues its alternating spikes signifying the chaotic and unproductive electrical activity going on in Harry's heart. The muscular nurse, at the instruction of the doctor, resumes compressions on the already fractured chest.

A well rehearsed series of medications are injected intravenously and several more shocks are administered to the shell that was Harry only twenty minutes ago. By now, even the wide eyed medical students realize that there is no more that can be done. Harry has completed his journey...alone in a hospital ICU.

Do you have a vision of what the end of your life will be? With some forethought and preparation the answer should be yes. Unlike taxes, the other universal truth in our society over which you have no direct control, your death and its conduct can be affected by choices that you make long before the last beat of your heart.

The intent of this book is to share experiences that I have had with patients and their families during what could have been very stressful times as life slipped away. My hope is that with some planning you may gain a feeling of control during your last days. Steps that you can take so that your death will be more peaceful and dignified with minimal anxiety, pain and existential suffering will be introduced through illustrative cases. I will alter details to

Bradley C. Buckhout, M.D.

protect patient confidentiality but the essence of the dilemmas and responses will be preserved to serve as points for discussion and education. This is a book based on medical issues and ultimately death and its conduct. I will endeavor to impart some of the humor and humanity that is present even in a field of medicine where death is the usual outcome and where our aim is to improve the quality of every remaining day and hour. A field where a "good death" is the ultimate goal, not the hastening of passing, but making the transition as gentle as possible for the patients and the people dear to them.

Death in America, indeed in the advanced countries of the world has become a medicalized event. The peace we all crave at the end is often replaced by futile medical procedures and medications provided by professionals who though well-intentioned are strangers and unaware of our desires and goals. Instead of expiring gently while reclining at home in a bed surrounded by family and well wishers the end for 56% of us occurs in a hospital and for another 19% in a nursing home.

This book, the culmination of thirty-nine years of medical experience will help you to consider your options for the last act of your life, an event that we will all face. It will hopefully be thought provoking enough that while you are of sound mind and in good health that you will reflect on the qualities of your existence that make your life meaningful and the compromises that you may be willing to make as your body begins to betray you. A series of important decisions need to be made, in advance, well before the final trip to the hospital and perhaps before considering that trip at all.

My experience as a physician began during a much simpler time in medicine and indeed in America. I began my medical school training in 1979 at the Medical College of Ohio at Toledo. There was no internet, no smartphones, no computerized medical records. CAT scans had not been introduced. When I needed to research a question, I went to the medical library and searched card catalogues for articles and chapters in text books for answers. As medical students we learned anatomy and physiology, the pathology of myriad disease processes. We were taught physical diagnosis skills, history taking and how to treat a wide array of conditions that would afflict our future patients.

We had a lecture describing the work of Elizabeth Kubler-Ross and the stages of grief. This was ground breaking work and paved the way for discussions that would make us all more sensitive to the steps that patients, families and indeed that we would go through when facing loss. But, Death was considered a defeat...a loss...a failure, something to be avoided at all costs. There were no lectures on caring for the dying. Palliative care, the choices that can be made to enhance the quality of the last days of a person's life and the final supportive philosophy of hospice care was not discussed.

My training after medical school continued in Toledo at the Mercy Hospital Family Medicine Residency Program. This program was the only full time residency at this inner city hospital. I chose this program as it would offer me the greatest exposure to patient care responsibility. In this period of medical training there were no hour limitations for residents and we, on call every third night, routinely worked 102 out of the possible 168 hours in a week. It was common to be making life and death decisions at 2 a.m. having been awake since 7 a.m. the day before. Times were different, our expectations were different. Medical care was much less technologically driven, we spent time talking with patients and saw them before ordering a battery of lab tests and x-rays...MRI's didn't exist. The tools and medications that we had at our disposal were, by today's standards, primitive.

Bradley C. Buckhout, M.D.

Medicine then was practiced with less intrusion by insurance and other third parties. It was a more personal, Dr. Marcus Welby style of care, when compassionate listening and time was as effective as the shot of B12 or penicillin given in the office .

The progress in the field of medicine has been astounding. Much of what I learned during my training has been replaced. Even the basic principles have been altered as refinements in our understanding of the human body, wellness and diseases mechanisms have been achieved. Medicine is a career that demands continual learning and the ability to adapt with the changing and ever expanding knowledge. Prior to enrolling in medical school I had a vision of the role that I would eventually play as a physician; I would become a family doctor.

Upon completion of training I moved my family to Arizona and opened a solo family medicine practice. My wife ran the office and our practice grew steadily over the twenty years that we worked together. We saw a diverse and largely healthy population of families. Newborns to centenarians were under our care whether they were in the office or hospitalized. Hospitalists didn't exist during the early years and I didn't accept them to care for "my" patients when they took over the hospitals. I spent hours in the operating room assisting surgeons with a wide variety of cases, something unheard of today and I made rounds on hospitalized patients in the early morning or in the evening after the office closed for the day.

Insurance company intrusion, declining reimbursement, time pressure to see more patients, increasing government regulations and deteriorating quality of life lead me to seek an alternate venue in which to continue to care for patients and we closed our practice after twenty years. A valued colleague with whom we had shared an office for half of that time suggested that I replace him following his retirement from the Department of Veterans Affairs. After some initial reservations I visited the Nursing Home Care Unit of our local VA and have had the honor of caring for our Nation's Veterans for the last sixteen years.

This has been an exceptionally challenging and rewarding endeavor focused on a largely geriatric patient population with many chronic health conditions. Preventative care opportunities are rare and managing chronic incurable conditions and complications are what occupies most of our time. As a result of caring for these patients, many of whom have a combination of conditions that are slowly but inexorably leading to their death, the emphasis and focus of my practice began to change again. In 2012 I became Board Certified in Hospice and Palliative Medicine, a new specialty first recognized in 1997.

Physicians who have chosen to practice palliative and hospice medicine are all board certified in another area primarily and have sought additional training to gain the specialized skills needed to work with the interdisciplinary team that cares for patients when curing is no longer an option. The American Board of Hospice & Palliative Medicine is the governing body that establishes the criteria to be met for the providers in this field and also is one of the bodies advocating for legislation to make the choices at the end of life more numerous.

Discussions concerning our options as life begins to ebb are thankfully becoming more commonplace. These conversations however, have become politically charged with discussions of government run death panels; religiously divisive with the oft repeated "slippery slope" concerns when either physician assisted suicide and euthanasia are mentioned and sensationalized by recounting the exploits of the late Dr. Jack Kevorkian. Palliative care and hospice support although dealing with the same

Bradley C. Buckhout, M.D.

patients are in truth not involved in any of these. There remains considerable confusion about the roles each of these specialties provide. Palliative care is a focus on the quality of life and truthfully should be considered much sooner for every patient. Who does not want to reduce suffering, improve function and increase enjoyment for every patient?

Medicine is big business, now consuming an estimated $3.4 trillion ($9596 per person) annually in the United States. Medicare figures show that 30% of the money spent goes for caring for the 5% of the members who will die that year and 1/3 of that total is spent in the last month. That might be acceptable if the quality of life were to be improved. Unfortunately, what those statistics suggest is that for many, the last days on this Earth are spent in a hospital enduring testing, procedures and treatments that do anything but enhance quality of life and many of which make the recipients miserable...with the same ultimate outcome.

Perhaps now is the appropriate time to share a parable that I learned from a mentor many years ago that applies to those for whom palliative care is appropriate...people with conditions that are no longer correctable, people who are going to die in the not too distant future despite the efforts of the many medical specialists intent on keeping them alive.

Two hikers are following a path through a remote jungle far from the nearest civilization. Suddenly, they are set upon by the warriors of a primitive tribe of head hunters. They are bound and taken at spear point to a clearing in the center of the head hunter village where they are lashed to elaborately carved poles positioned within ear shot but out of sight of each other. Hearts pounding loudly in their ears they wait, fear building as the number of menacing villagers grows as word of the new arrivals spreads.

When Caring Trumps Curing

Finally, as the sun reaches its peak overhead an imposing man wearing an elaborate headdress and a necklace of shrunken heads strides with obvious authority from his tent and approaches the first hiker. After inspecting her carefully, he sneers, "Death or Che-Che?"

She begins to whimper, "How can I answer, I don't know what that is?"

He approaches more closely, his gaze boring into her tearful eyes while slowly withdrawing a dagger from his belt and repeats, "Death or Che-Che? Choose!"

"I don't...Oh, please, why? I can't decide!" The dagger point rises slowly toward her and she cries out, "Che-Che".

At this, the Chief plunges the dagger into the post above her head and steps back as she is swarmed over by the warriors all armed with similar blades. Her screams pierce the jungle and after several minutes she mercifully falls silent, her blood and life drained from her.

Across the clearing, her companion has been a witness to the sound of what has happened but he has no idea what has befallen his friend. His heart is racing as he struggles to breathe expecting that he is next. His mind races, he struggles against the ropes that hold him fast to his pole. He does not know what Che-Che is but he does not want to experience its horrifying results.

The Chief, spattered with blood suddenly appears in front of him his hideous grin exposing his discolored, crooked teeth. He approaches and poses the feared question, "Death or Che-Che?"

Bradley C. Buckhout, M.D.

Thinking that Death may be the lesser evil of the options with which he is presented he hesitates but gasps, "death..."

The Chief, his grin broadening replies, "Ah yes...but first a little Che-Che."

Chapter 2
Medical Advances

There is a time in every life when the force to continue is so weak that nothing will be able to reinvigorate the body to live on. Unfortunately, modern medicine has such an impressive array of tools to beat back death that it is almost impossible to get to the point where we have run out of things to be done to a patient. One of the philosophical principals that drives palliative care is the statement to a patient, "there is always something more that can be done to you…the question is, is it being done for you?"

Medical advances over the last century have occurred at a prodigious rate and have changed expectations about when someone is likely to die and of what cause. In the early 1900's, death was most commonly attributed to infections: influenza/pneumonia, tuberculosis, diarrhea and enteritis as there were no antibiotics and sanitation and public health were not well developed concepts. People in the U.S. lived to an average age of 46 years. When they became ill there was little that could be done, therapies were limited and ineffective. Doctors, when they were consulted at all came to the home and sat at the bedside comforting the patient and the family as the disease process continued to its completion. The care being provided was supportive and focused on palliation of symptoms.

In 1928 Alexander Fleming accidentally discovered the anti-staphylococcal properties of a mold, Penicillium. Progress was slow on developing this life changing breakthrough and penicillin was not used to treat patients until 1942. Sulfa was identified as having antibacterial properties in 1935 and was used to great

Bradley C. Buckhout, M.D.

benefit in World War II battlefield wounds and later in the civilian population, changing the dynamics of acute illness and mortality. With these miracles, the most common causes of death changed to heart disease, lung disease and cancers and the average age at death increased to approximately 60 years. The rapidly progressive infections that had caused the deaths of many previously healthy people were now being cured by the discovery of these effective treatments. Chronic conditions such as heart disease, lung disease and cancers began their dominance of our morbidity and mortality. Early in the century the understanding of the mechanisms leading to these conditions were poorly understood. Doctors proclaimed the health benefits of certain brands of cigarettes, dietary fat was not the enemy that it eventually became, no one "exercised"; work provided enough physical activity.

When people became ill, they more readily sought medical care and frequently were hospitalized, sometimes to their benefit. When I began my medical training in the late 1970's however, it was still not uncommon for patients being admitted to the hospital to freely admit that since they were ill enough to need hospitalization, they were likely never going to see their home again.

During the last forty years the advances have been astonishing. Information technology (computers, the internet, smart phones); imaging (CAT scans, MRI's, angiography, PET scans); therapies (coronary and peripheral arterial bypass and stents, laparoscopic surgeries, robot assisted surgery, radiation therapy, gamma knife surgery, organ transplantation) and medications (antibiotics by the score, cardiac meds, statins, anti-HIV drugs, chemotherapy agents, immune modulating biologics) to name only a small sampling, have all had huge impacts on the care of patients. Life expectancy has increased from 68 years to an average of 78 years during this period and the general perception is that death is not an inevitable outcome of illness.

People encouraged by the successes of the medical profession and the pharmaceutical industry have the expectation that their ills can be cured and if not cured, then managed successfully extending life. A favorite cartoon shows a patient seated in the doctors office with the doctor proclaiming, "...any quack therapy can make you feel better for a while, but only modern medicine can keep you alive forever."

The advances in care have lead to the medicalization of many conditions that were previously thought not amenable to drug therapy. We are bombarded with direct to consumer advertising for medications to treat everything from diabetes to erectile dysfunction, non-24 sleep disorder, small cell lung cancer. Death has become not an inevitable result of life, but a foe that can be defeated with the proper medication regimen, diet or surgical treatment. This is apparent when it is noted that 40% of Americans believe that medical technology can always save their lives!

The internet as a source of unverified and unfiltered information has fostered some of these optimistic and unrealistic expectations. Television dramas based in hospitals have failed to provide realistic portrayals of pretty much everything related to the practice of medicine. At least once an episode someone rolls into the emergency department after a cardiac arrest and is quickly resuscitated, gets dressed and heads home to finish mowing the lawn, the activity he was performing at the time of his collapse. These shows have fostered the belief in the absolute power of medical care and that death can be dealt a fatal blow when applied by the young attractive intern who has just learned that the chief of surgery is her long lost father.

Bradley C. Buckhout, M.D.

As we enter a new phase of immuno-biology in which drugs are being created utilizing the body's immune mechanisms targeted specifically against the antigens that are present on the cancer cells growing within, we will be moving towards changing the dynamics of cancer and its' relationship to dying. It is becoming apparent that cancer, like AIDS will soon become another chronic disease to be managed similar to other incurable but manageable conditions like arthritis, diabetes, copd, hypertension and others. The unfortunate corollary to this is the aging American's social calendar will be filled with appointments to the multiple medical practitioners that will be required to monitor his growing problem list.

The well trained family practitioner will be an ideal resource for managing these ever more complicated patients. Someone in concert with the patient needs to be the captain of this complex ship as it navigates the risks of the uncharted waters of these new disease management regimens. As medical providers, one of our more vital tasks is to educate our patients about the diseases they face, the options in treatments that can be offered and the likely benefits and costs of each. The days of medical paternalism have expired. Informed consent is the concept that drives the decision making for care today. But one must acknowledge that much of the information that is available is incomplete and not well understood and that often the advice that we provide is based on an optimistic projection of what is to come, targeted to a patient with a fund of medical knowledge which is inadequate for the task.

Maintenance of Independence is the phrase heard most often as people age and are asked what is the most important thing to them. It is rare to hear a wish to live as long as possible. Some people have specific goals in mind: "to make it to our 50th wedding anniversary"; "he has to be there to walk our daughter down the aisle at her wedding"; "my granddaughter is graduating from college in the spring". What seniors fear the most is losing independence, the isolation of the inability to drive; having to move from the house that has been a home for decades; needing the assistance of a stranger to manage the previously simple tasks known as the activities of daily living.

As medical care becomes more successful the term elderly continually is being reassessed. At what age does one become a senior citizen? It depends on who is defining this milestone. Movie theaters give a break at 60, Medicare eligibility is slowly creeping up from 65 to 66+ based on the year of birth. I have seen hip replacements for arthritis being done to patients in their mid 80's. This would not have been considered when I began practicing. One hears 60 is the new 40. We can all hope that this is true and that advances in care will continue with one very large caveat. The quantity of life may not be the most important goal for which we should strive. To live to a ripe old age, perhaps even crossing the century mark while being confined to bed in an institution with a variety of supportive medical devices, care givers who are at best well meaning strangers and with little comprehension of one's surroundings or purpose is a fate that is facing a growing number of our elderly. Dementia in all of its cruel varieties continues to add victims to its rolls despite the commercials reassuring us that a cure will be here during our lifetime.

This brings me to one of the most important reasons for this book. It is a plea to the reader, no matter where you are in the journey of your life, to begin to consider some very important decisions that will guide you and your loved ones as the end of your voyage approaches. There are few of us alive now who will die suddenly. Certainly accidents, particularly motor vehicle caused deaths are in the news often but statistics show that in 2015 the rate was 1.13 fatalities for every 100 million miles driven.

Bradley C. Buckhout, M.D.

The leading cause of death, cardiac disease also may manifest as a sudden event with 424,000 cardiac arrests occurring in 2014. Often this sudden collapse is the first indication of the underlying disease and survival details are not very encouraging. Most of these events occur at home (69%). When witnessed and emergency medical services are summoned the survival rate is 10%. In a situation where the collapse is witnessed and cardiopulmonary resuscitation is started before the EMS team arrives (with defibrillator use by the public when available) the survival of the event is 31%. One would think that being in the hospital at the time of a cardiac arrest would be of benefit. Not so much. The hospital arrest victim survives only 16% of the time. On considering these numbers, the contradiction of better survival from a witnessed non-hospitalized event would initially seem illogical. But one must consider that the patient in the hospital was already seriously ill enough to require hospital admission and the out of hospital arrest victim may have been a relatively healthy younger male (almost always), whose first presentation of his cardiac disease is an arrhythmia that would otherwise be fatal without the intervention of bystanders and EMS personnel.

The term survival in these statistics means the victim was eventually discharged from the hospital alive. However, an additional alarming piece of news is that neurologic function was considered "good" in only 8.3% of those who were alive on discharge. This means there was significant brain function loss during the period that the heart was not beating effectively. The common location for discharge for these unlucky souls is a long term care facility (a politically correct euphemism for a nursing home).

So barring the rare event when life is suddenly extinguished and knowing that advances in medicine are approaching the Holy Grail of "Keeping you Alive Forever" the important question you must begin to contemplate is, "would I want this?" This is not a question to be taken lightly, perhaps not even a question that you can answer strictly by yourself if you are fortunate enough to have significant people in your life who care about you. The answer to this question has many layers and will, for most people, require some time to formulate an answer that is correct for you. The answer will need to be revisited as your life situation changes, you mature and your health issues begin to mount and as your view of the future evolves.

What features of your existence make your life meaningful? What are the qualities of your life that make waking each day an experience that you anticipate with hope and enthusiasm? What is it about each day that provides pleasure and your reason for being? Do you handle adversity and challenge with a commitment to persevere and conquer or with dread and pessimism? The answer to these questions can then be extended to what qualities of your life, if lost would make your life not worth living? What functions, relationships, abilities could you lose and still view your life as worthy of continuing? What could you not tolerate? To what ends would you go to preserve your life, would it depend on the quality of life that remains or would you want to stay alive as long as medically possible?

As we age, there is a good probability that we will acquire medical conditions that will slowly erode our abilities to carry out our routine activities, impair our memory or other important cognitive functions or will lead to pain or disability which may take us to the point of being dependent on others for our care. Unfortunately, in America the traditional nuclear family and location stability has faded. People are mobile, families are scattered across the country and even the globe and the tradition of the elders of the family being cared for by the younger members is a rarity today. There is a growing number of single person households, particularly among woman over 75 yrs of age, almost half of whom are living alone, but also in younger people 27% of whom reside by themselves. To whom will they turn when they are no longer able to live alone? Friends will be challenged to provide care and will soon be overwhelmed by the burden. If you were alone to whom would you turn?

To assist you in answering these questions, I would like to introduce in the next chapter several resources that can assist by providing guidance, some terms that you may have heard but about which you may be unclear and perhaps also pose some alternatives that had not occurred to you.

Chapter 3
Advanced Care Planning

Advanced directives, living wills, medical powers of attorney, competency, capacity, code status (DNR or resuscitate) are all topics for which clarification may be helpful to aid in your deliberations. A Google search of "advanced directives" returned over 27,000,000 sites, clearly a need has been discovered! There are abundant sources that offer assistance for creating legal advanced care planning documents. Some of the information is state specific, some can be applied universally across the country and there are a multitude of foreign sources as well.

All states have statutes called advanced directives or health care directives that allow their citizens to make future health care treatment decisions at their convenience. Then, if an incapacitating illness occurs later, medical providers and family will know what treatments are desired and which should not be considered. These laws also allow for the selection of a representative to make end of life decisions, or more precisely to relay the wishes previously enumerated by the now incapacitated individual.

Since my work most recently has been caring for our nation's veterans, I am most familiar with the Life Sustaining Treatment Decision Initiative, a product of the National Center for Ethics in Healthcare. (See Appendix A) This organization provides study and guidance for ethical care of the veteran population in the VA system. Other healthcare organizations, insurers, government and advocacy groups are developing similar programs to address the very important topic of advanced care planning.

Bradley C. Buckhout, M.D.

The starting point for this important process is the Goals of Care Conversation. At present this is most often carried out in the hospital when some critical illness requires urgent life or death decisions to be made. It is most often initiated by a medical provider, hopefully trained in the techniques of this sometimes emotional discussion. The vision for this process is that these conversations will eventually be introduced by a patient's own provider in an office visit under much less stressful conditions with time for reflection and deliberation. After reading this book perhaps you will be the one to initiate the subject and will feel comfortable laying out your plans and desires for your final chapter.

How does one begin? When is the "right time" to have these conversations? As mentioned above, changing conditions and situations may dictate the timing; a diagnosis of cancer, mental slipping signaling the onset of dementia, frailty and declining independence, loss of a loved one all should trigger thoughts of clarifying the goals of care. In a later chapter, a case will give an example of the goals of care discussion and may serve as a model for a thoughtful review of your wishes for the future.

A recent conversation with a couple whose elderly mother has been stricken with dementia reinforced the need for more information as we all plan for the inevitable end. "You mean there is more than just DNR that we need to consider?" The simple answer is yes, much more. You have the power, if you know the questions, to prepare for unsuspected eventualities and complications that may occur. I first would like to provide some explanations for terms that you will often hear to help you negotiate the maze of possibilities.

Advanced Directives or Health Care Directives or Living Will:

When Caring Trumps Curing

These are legal documents that allow us to make future health care treatment decisions now so that at some future date when incapacitation has taken the ability to make decisions our families and doctors will know what we want and don't want. As a medical provider, I have seen many poorly executed advanced directives with responses to a variety of questions "it depends" with no qualification. This is completely useless and provides no direction at a time when critical decisions must be made. As you are considering your options, being as specific as possible is very helpful to those providing your care when time may be of the essence. Clear statements also relieve your family members and designated surrogates with clear direction of your intentions and desires.

I would like to provide, as an example, statements from a well thought out living will:

1. If I have a terminal condition, I DO NOT want my life prolonged and I DO NOT want life-sustaining treatment, beyond comfort care, that would only serve to prolong the moment of my death.

2. If I am in an irreversible coma or persistent vegetative state, a terminal condition that doctors feel is incurable, I DO want medical care to keep me comfortable, but I DO NOT want the following:
    a. Cardiopulmonary resuscitation (including drugs, electric shocks and artificial respiration).
    b. Artificially administered food and fluids.
    c. To be taken to a hospital if it can be avoided.

In addition to these basic statements, an addendum to this document has been included:

Bradley C. Buckhout, M.D.

1. Upon admission to an intensive care unit whether by transfer from an inpatient hospital unit or directly from the emergency department, I direct the attending physician to obtain a consultation with a palliative care specialist.

2. If I require intubation and ventilator support for a condition felt to be reversible, I consent to the use of this device, however if my condition has not improved and tracheostomy is being considered, I consent only if the palliative care team agrees that this action is not just prolonging my death.

3. If I can no longer swallow effectively, I do not consent to the placement of a PEG (percutaneous feeding tube) or nasogastric/duotube feeding devices.

4. In the event of a terminal diagnosis, the focus of care is to be on quality of life and not prolonging the dying process.

The other important document to accompany your advanced directives is one that designates your trusted decision maker if you are incapacitated. The choice of this person, someone who will reliably act on your behalf, is also a decision to be carefully considered. Your durable power of attorney for healthcare is given to the person that you trust to make medical decisions for you in an emergency. Even though you have been fairly inclusive and explicit in your living will, there may occur situations which you have not considered and therefore not addressed and your medical power of attorney gives your designee (surrogate decision maker, proxy, advocate, agent, attorney-in-fact) the legal authority to make decisions for you. Keep in mind, the person with your durable medical power of attorney cannot contradict the terms of your living will. They are to fill in the gaps not covered in the documents that you have completed and would provide guidance if the living will was invalidated for some reason. In their role, they have the right to enforce your wishes in court if needed. They may hire and fire physicians caring for you and have access to the medical records and have the privilege of visitation rights.

It is worth spending a little time discussing this very important designation. The person you finally elect may not be the person you would first consider as your spokesperson. The person that you choose should be someone in whom you have the utmost confidence to understand and embrace your wishes. Difficult decisions may very likely need to be made at the end of your life and you want your designee to be a strong advocate for <u>your</u> wishes. There are many things to consider and discussions with your spouse, significant other, children, friends and/or professionals may be required to prevent painful emotionally charged battles down the road.

I have been involved in too many cases during which the wishes of the patient are forgotten because the surrogate's emotions take over and they substitute their judgment and their inability to let go with the desires of the patient (often a parent or spouse). Considering this, perhaps one of your children, the analytical first child perhaps, would be a better person to hold your fate as opposed to the emotionally labile youngest child who will under no circumstances stop any medical intervention even long after it is clear that the opportunity for benefit has passed. As couples age together, it is common for them to serve this role for each other. But after many years together the final decision to allow death to occur is the last loving act that is often very difficult to perform.

If we revisit for a moment the elderly couple that were introduced in the first chapter, Harry and Vivian, several scenarios can be constructed to explain how Harry came to such a traumatic end, alone in an ICU at the moment of his death. Hopefully, he and Vivian had discussions about what he would have wanted when his heart finally gave out. Despite all of the obvious signs that he was beginning a steep decline in his health and that he was unlikely going to live to their next anniversary, there is no evidence in this vignette that he had requested a do not resuscitate order. Had his cardiologist spent time with the two of them explaining that the weapons remaining were becoming impotent to combat the ongoing deterioration of the heart muscle? Had there been a consultation with the palliative care team who would have encouraged a frank assessment of what was important to Harry and his wife? Had everyone avoided the inevitability of the end approaching with plans to talk about this later?

Our population is aging and as a consequence there are increasing numbers of elderly members of our society with dementia in all of its cruel forms. Recent estimates suggest 5.5 million Americans over the age of 65 (10% of this age group) and an additional 200,000 younger than 65 years are afflicted. Dementia is not a sudden event and hopefully the senior members of our society have made appropriate plans for their future medical care. This is less likely in the younger group as the "sense of indestructibility gene" has not yet withered completely in this age group.

This brings up two additional terms for discussion, competency and capacity. Competency is a legal term referring to the mental ability and cognitive capabilities required to execute a legally recognized act rationally. The determination of incompetence is a judicial decision, i.e., decided by the court. An individual adjudicated by the court as incompetent is referred to as de jure incompetent.

Capacity is also a legal term evaluating the ability of a person to act on his/her own behalf. The ability to understand information presented, to appreciate the consequences of acting or not acting on that information and to be able to make a choice is evidence of capacity. This assessment is often completed by medical providers using clinical assessments of the patient and sometimes includes specific cognitive testing when the answer is unclear. Capacity in the medical arena may be applied to specific questions and situations. For instance it may be clear that a patient no longer has the capacity to live independently, that he does not have sufficient understanding and memory to comprehend in a general way the situation in which he finds himself and the nature, purpose, and consequence of any act or transaction into which he might enter. But in the immediate situation he may be able to comprehend the nature of his illness and the consequence of either accepting or rejecting the treatments that are being planned and to make a choice consistent with his known values and beliefs.

Does the person have the mental capacity to make decisions about life sustaining treatments? In other words, can the patient understand his condition and the consequences of choosing to accept or decline treatments being offered. As an example, if he chooses to not have cardiac resuscitation attempted, does he realize that he will die? If the answer to this question is "no", the person lacks capacity. The important question that then needs to be answered, who is the surrogate decision maker? Hopefully, previously completed advanced directives will answer this question. If not, there is a state specific hierarchy of persons to assume this role. This will be addressed more fully in a later chapter but is another good reason to consider and complete your documents now, while you have control of your faculties and this important choice. In Arizona the progression is spouse, adult children with no specific order specified and often a source of inter-sibling

Bradley C. Buckhout, M.D.

conflict. In the case of conflict, majority rules with the physician as the tie breaker. Next are parents, domestic partner, siblings (see above for conflict resolution), close friend who perhaps knows more about the wishes of the patient than estranged family. In the situation where none of these exist and there is no advanced directive, the attending physician in consultation with the ethics committee or if none exists, a second physician will make decisions in the best interest of the patient from their medical perspective.

As an example, a veteran who was afflicted with ALS (Amyotrophic Lateral Sclerosis) a cruel, eventually fatal neurodegenerative disease was admitted to the intensive care unit due to respiratory failure. He was intubated to keep him breathing and required placement of a tube into his stomach for nutritional support. He was eventually unable to communicate and was not apparently aware of his surroundings but his wife, who threatened legal action against the hospital if he was transferred from the ICU, caused him to remain alive for 4 1/2 years before he finally succumbed. He had no advanced directive despite his medical condition with its poor prognosis and so had no say in how and where he passed the last years of his life.

All adults should have an advance directive!

When Americans are asked where they would like to be for their last days, the overwhelming response (80%) is at home. The actual location of death, far too often is in a hospital (56%) or a nursing home (19%) with death at home occurring only 20% of the time. When you consider this question, what do you desire? Are you a never give up, fight to the end, win at any cost, stay alive despite substantial functional losses kind of person? If these are your wishes then perhaps ending your life with intravenous lines, foley catheters, oxygen delivery equipment, confined in a hospital bed is acceptable to you. If this is the case, be certain that you have specified this to the person who will instruct the medical team when you are unable to communicate any longer.

If you believe that comfort can be found at home, in familiar surroundings with your music and books, pets at your bedside being attended to by your family and perhaps visiting hospice nurses, then this needs to be expressed clearly as well. Once at home, there are documents available that should also be completed that will relieve the paramedics of the obligation to do things to you that you no longer find appropriate or necessary. Physician Order for Life-Sustaining Treatment (POLST) Form: This is called different things in different states (e.g., MOLST, MOST, POST) regardless of the term, a POLST Form is a medical order for the specific medical treatments you want during a medical emergency. Individuals with a serious illness or advanced frailty near the end-of-life should have this form. People being cared for by a hospice agency will have this form or something similar.

POLST (Physician Orders for Life Sustaining Treatment) form, is helpful for out of hospital direction for care givers and is a legal order for the care to be provided or more specifically to be withheld. Without this form or something similar (in Arizona the "Orange Form"), first responders are obligated to begin resuscitation until directed by a higher medical authority to cease. This form is the medical authority on which they can rely for this decision to prevent the trauma to your body implicit in CPR.

The Arizona Orange Form so called because it MUST be printed on orange paper is formally titled the "Prehospital Medical Care Directive (Do Not Resuscitate)". It is affixed to the refrigerator of the residence and identifies the patient for whom it applies. It states: "In the event of cardiac or respiratory arrest, I refuse any resuscitation measures including cardiac compression, endotracheal intubation and other advanced airway management, artificial ventilation, defibrillation, administration of advanced cardiac life support drugs and related emergency medical procedures."

The patient signs the document and identifies their physician and/or hospice organization. The provider also signs the document as does a notary or witness. The forms vary from state to state and all states have not fully adopted this program so you will need to check with your health care provider for what is available where you live.

See Appendix B

This chapter has hopefully clarified some of the confusing terminology associated with end of life care and planning. We will now move on to several illustrative cases which will present choices and consequences for these specific patients. Nothing in medicine is completely generalizable, but each case was chosen for its lessons from which we can all benefit.

PART 2

Chapter 4
The Price of Freedom is Visible Here

As I mentioned in the first chapter of this book, my career in medicine has evolved during decades of marvelous medical development and changes in our culture medically and as a society. The constant has been change. Even after four decades of practice, I am on a weekly basis still seeing things that I have never previously encountered. The obvious need to continually upgrade knowledge and to keep an open mind to remain abreast of the advances is apparent nearly every day. My medical career began as a traditional solo family practitioner with my wife manning the front office and serving in the roles normally occupied by at least three staff members in larger offices, a medical assistant with me in the back and a part time student helping with the filing. We served generations of families from newborn to great-great-grandmas. It was a largely healthy population, deaths were rare and in my twenty years only one patient required the amputation of a gangrenous limb.

The transition from this autonomous practice model to the largest health care organization in the country, the Department of Veterans Affairs was a move that I was not initially considering. So, why one might ask, would I close my private practice to become a physician in a VA Nursing Home? Initially, out of respect for my former partner who was soon to retire from the VA, I went for a visit and immediately realized that this place would be a pleasant change. I would be able to escape the

Bradley C. Buckhout, M.D.

crushing hours that my wife and I were putting in everyday and still be able to focus on providing excellent patient care, now to the veterans of our country's military.

In stark contrast to my isolation as a solo practitioner, the support from multiple other medical specialists and diagnostic services, professionals in nursing, pharmacy, physical and occupational therapy, psychology, social work, chaplaincy and recreation therapy were readily available. I joined other physicians and mid-level providers (nurse practitioners and physician assistants) in the nursing home as a team to care for the patients. There was evidence of a caring dedication for the veterans apparent every day. This practice allowed time for interactions with the veterans and their families that was beyond simple medical care and as I think back, the philosophy of palliative care was already being incorporated in the functioning of the nursing home care unit.

Physicians assume many roles when caring for patients, one of the most important is that of educator. As a family doctor, I spent countless hours explaining to patients what specialists had not clearly described; test results, procedures planned, treatment recommendations and even prognosis for serious life threatening illnesses. In exchange for my educating them, patients have taught me many things about hope, faith, resilience, courage, love and the search for meaning and purpose in this life.

I have spent time at the bedside, comforting men who served in Africa in World War II, who survived the attack at Pearl Harbor, who landed on the beaches of Normandy, survived German POW camps, tramped through the jungles of Vietnam bathed by Agent Orange, served on submarines and carriers off the coast of that country and who flew missions in aircraft over Southeast Asia. The stories that they have shared have given meaning and life to the withered, aged bodies that are brought to our unit near the end of their remarkable journeys.

The stories of these American veterans are difficult for civilians to comprehend but many similar accounts have been published and memorialized in film. They are important for all Americans to know as they demonstrate the dedication and sacrifice that our fellow citizens have made for the benefit of all of us back home. We have a mural on the wall at the entrance to our unit, "The Price of Freedom is Visible Here". It truly is and it has been an honor to care for these men and women.

I would like to share with you some of the stories of the patients for whom I have provided care for the purpose of clarifying some of what the first part of the book described. These cases are all unique patient experiences but they all have some universal truths, dilemmas and resolutions that are widely applicable and may help you with your planning and decisions for the future. The patients are all real. I have changed the names and some of the details to obscure identities and preserve patient privacy without making this a work of fiction. In discussing the cases, I will expand some of the discussions to include options and alternatives that were not chosen by the patient/family but that will add to your understanding of the choices that you may consider.

Bradley C. Buckhout, M.D.

Chapter 5
EMIL

Every large family seems to have that one unusual uncle, the one who comes to Christmas dinner wearing the green elf shoes with the curling toes adorned by the little silver bells that tinkle merrily as they skip into the family gathering singing Jingle Bells...off key of course. Ours was Uncle Emil. He would travel each year from his beachside home in South Carolina to our home in Eau Claire, Wisconsin, that in itself perhaps a clue to his degree of sanity.

Uncle Emil had served in the Navy from the end of World War II through the Korean conflict as a radio operator. He had become a musician, entrepreneur, comedian. He was semi-successful except in relationships which were not amenable to his travels and sketchy finances. Near his home in Myrtle Beach, he had become a regular, performing his guitar enhanced comedy routine at The Sandy Crab, overlooking the breakers of the Atlantic. He attracted the attention of the college kids on Spring Break with his bawdy lyrical creations to familiar songs. On one of his trips to Eau Claire at Christmas he brought his guitar to entertain the family and one evening went to an open mic night at O'Leary's Pub near the Eau Claire campus of the University of Wisconsin. The college crowd there went crazy and he was offered a permanent gig on the spot. He agreed for the spring and summer in Wisconsin and then would return to his other job in the winter at the beach...maybe he wasn't so crazy after all.

"Do a shot with Emil" became a mainstay of his performances. If an audience member could sing the next line of the song Emil was playing he won a shot of tequila, if not Emil gulped the shot. Some nights his crowd wasn't very good and the performance deteriorated to the delight of the college crowd as Emil consumed his 13th shot for the evening. After several years of his cross country commuting, an accident in Myrtle Beach involving a car load of students who had been very good at singing along and who should not have been driving nearly killed the driver and a person in the other car. Uncle Emil took stock of his health and the effect that his act was having on him and also felt a deep sense of responsibility for nearly causing the deaths of several inebriated youths and he acted. He stopped drinking and soon after stopped his forty year smoking habit. We remained in contact over the next several years and after I graduated from Marquette with a business degree and began my real estate investing firm I sought advice from Uncle Emil. I was unfamiliar with the economy of South Carolina but suspected coastal development to be a potentially lucrative market for my firm. Emil helped me with contacts and he actually began to devote time to promote my company and found me my first condo investment property.

Over the last eight years, he has gradually given up his career in entertainment. He blames the progressive deformity of his arthritic fingers which makes playing the guitar painfully difficult. He won't admit it, but I think it is largely due to his desire for his favorite nephew's business to succeed. My company thankfully, is growing quite nicely and I felt it was partly due to Uncle Emil's encouragement and contacts. So five years ago, I began to pay him a salary to manage my office in Myrtle Beach when I was home in Wisconsin.

Two years ago while I was vacationing in Costa Rica, I happened upon a multistory condo overlooking the Pacific in Playas del Coco. The price was right and the transaction was surprisingly easy, so Wisconsin Beaches Realty took ownership and I installed Uncle Emil as the complex manager. He had been living there full time, stretched out in his beach chair watching the sun

Bradley C. Buckhout, M.D.

disappear into the ocean each evening. We spoke by phone regularly and rendezvoused on occasion in Arizona so that he could keep me updated on the state of our international investment. All was going well. Emil was enjoying his new location and the job was not too demanding. As always, he had quickly developed a cadre of new friends; life was good.

It is hard to believe that it was only four months ago with all that has transpired but I guess it's true...I still can't quite believe he's gone. I wasn't there for the beginning of the story but Emil filled me in the night I picked him up at Sky Harbor Airport. I almost didn't recognize the slumped pale old man that the attendant rolled out to my car in a wheelchair that night. I was shocked that a man that tanned could look so ghostly pale!

Two weeks earlier he had started having some night sweats, not uncommon for the tropics, but he had chills as well. He quickly grew progressively more fatigued so that a doze in a hammock at the beach became a nearly daylong slumber. When he set off on his usual two mile walk along the beach, he was only able to make it to the next condo down the beach before having to stop and rest and it was then a struggle to make it back home.

Guys tend to stubbornly ignore illness presuming that it will get better with time until they are grabbed by the proverbial throat with a shout in the ear, "WAKE UP! There's something wrong!" For Emil his moment was when he got up in the middle of the night to head for the bathroom and passed out. When he awoke with a bloody nose he decided to seek medical attention. The local doctor, to his credit, got a CBC (a blood sample which measures hemoglobin, white blood cells and platelet count). The only thing Uncle Emil could remember was his white count was high, in the neighborhood of fifty-thousand. The doctor, trying to make sense of the lab and his patient's story presumed he had an infection and gave him an injection of rocephin, a broad spectrum antibiotic and instructed rest and a follow up appointment on Monday morning.

Emil complied but continued to get weaker and the chills at night continued. He began to get concerned and asked one of his tenants and new found friends to drive him to the CIMA hospital satellite in Liberia, the nearest city in the Guanacaste province. The main hospital has an agreement with the United States VA and is also affiliated with Baylor University so the emergency room was staffed by well trained physicians who recognized that Uncle Emil's white blood count of 101,600 was not due to an infection and along with the other symptoms pointed to something far more serious. The doctor recommended immediate admission to the hospital but Emil wanted to be admitted to a hospital in the States and that is when he called me. Thankfully, I was at my apartment in Phoenix and I readily agreed to meet him at the airport and to transport him to the hospital if he could get himself to the plane in Costa Rica.

After I gathered Uncle Emil and lifted him from the wheelchair provided by the SkyCap into my car and tossed his bag into the trunk, we headed out of the airport for the freeway and the nearest hospital.

"Dick, you'll need to take me to the VA. I don't have any other health insurance," he said almost inaudibly.

"What do you mean you don't have health insurance Uncle Emil, you are old enough for Medicare?"

"I didn't get around to applying, so I don't know if I have coverage…I'm a veteran and I've been to the VA before, they'll take care of me."

Bradley C. Buckhout, M.D.

Thankfully, the VA was not far. Uncle Emil was looking bad enough that when the attendant with the wheelchair helped him from the car, we bypassed several other veterans languishing uncomfortably in the waiting room. Soon after the intake nurse had taken his vitals and had entered his recent history, as incomplete as it was, into the computer a tech showed up and drew another CBC along with some other tests. This time, less than 22 hours since the last one in Liberia, the white blood cells had climbed to an even more alarming 342,000. As a comparison for non-medical persons the normal white count is 4,500 to 10,000. This number of white blood cells is seen only in acute leukemia.

Uncle Emil was immediately transferred to the University Medical Center for aggressive management of his leukemia. This many white cells increase the blood viscosity and leads to stasis of blood in the small vessels impairing oxygen delivery to the tissues causing damage to organs such as the heart, brain, gut, kidneys and liver. Because the bone marrow has been commandeered by the neoplastic cells, the production of red cells and platelets declines so that severe anemia and bleeding episodes are common.

Leukopharesis, or removal of white blood cells by a process similar to dialysis was started immediately and was followed by induction chemotherapy with cytarabine and daunorubicin. These medications, like many traditional anti-cancer drugs nonselectively damage any cells that are rapidly reproducing. The goal of the treatment is to kill the cancer cells which are reproducing at such a high rate that they threaten the survival of the body they are inhabiting. The disease and the treatment caused a precipitous decline in Uncle Emil's kidney function. A large IV line had to be placed in his neck so that dialysis could be started to support his failing kidneys during the initiation of treatment for this rare cancer. The bone marrow biopsy that had been taken on the first day came back confirming acute myelogenous leukemia. This malignancy occurs more commonly in those over 65 years of age but is relatively rare and causes only 1.2% of the annual cancer deaths in the United States. Uncle Emil, at 71 years of age, had a difficult course ahead and statistically only a 5-15% chance for a cure, if he could tolerate the aggressive chemotherapy.

His condition following the chemo infusion deteriorated further. He writhed in bed from the severe piercing, cramping abdominal pain which was only partially relieved by forceful vomiting and bouts of watery diarrhea. His white count plunged to less than 1000 putting him at risk for infections and his hemoglobin dropped to less than 6 gms requiring transfusions.

Dialysis took 4 hours out of every other day to control the fluid levels and to remove the waste products in his blood. He would sleep during the run and then was so exhausted on return that he slept most of the day. He couldn't eat due to the vomiting and abdominal pain and I could see him shrinking steadily when I came to sit by his bedside to try to distract and comfort him.

"Dick, I'm sorry but I think the treatment is killing me faster than the disease...I don't think I can do this again," he said between wretches and spitting into his emesis basin.

"Have you talked to your doctors Uncle Emil, do they know what you're thinking?"

"Not yet, I know they are trying hard and I don't want to disappoint them. I wanted to talk with you first so that I can come to some decisions...I need you to be my spokesman...Dick, you are my closest family and I trust you to have my best interest at heart should I not be able to express myself."

Bradley C. Buckhout, M.D.

As presented in Part I of this book, designating a surrogate decision maker for you as your body begins to suggest more directly that your days may be numbered is of great importance. Without the directions that you specify in an advanced directive document or in a life sustaining treatment discussion with a provider, you may be subjected to continuation of life preserving interventions that as Emil said make you feel like you wish the end would come sooner. You should discuss your wishes, your goals, the treatments that you might accept and those that you want to avoid with your surrogate. They must have a clear understanding of your opinion as to what constitutes the important qualities of you and your existence. They need to know that when those key components are irretrievably lost that it is time to stop trying to cure and to change to a palliative focus.
This is a time when caring trumps curing!

After conversations with the oncologist and the nephrologist, the University Medical Center palliative care team was called and they sat with Emil and me and we reviewed the course of his disease, the likely outcomes if he continued with therapy and for the first time, the option of not continuing therapy. Along with the second option they discussed the dreaded "H" word; hospice. I think we all have a picture of what we think hospice means: death. How many times have we heard, they called in hospice and she died three days later?

Author's Note: I agree that this perception is common, but as a palliative and hospice physician, my interpretation is opposite of that of the general public. Rather than hospice being the cause of the patient's death, it is a clear sign that the consult to the hospice service was made much too late in the course of the disease. Hospice care givers are, by their nature, dedicated to providing comfort to patients and families as they transition from this life to whatever comes after. It is unfortunate that their services are not utilized in the last months of life rather than in the precious few days or hours at the very end.

I watched Uncle Emil as the palliative team began to explain the meaning, the purpose, the philosophy of hospice care. His face registered initial fear, disbelief and then as he heard more he relaxed and I could see relief as his eyes filled with tears.

It had been twenty-eight days since Uncle Emil left the hammock lazily swinging over the sand on the beach in Costa Rica, his guitar cradled across his chest as he strummed and sang …. 'strumming my six string on my front porch swing…smell those shrimp, hey they're beginning to boil…' and now we were headed for Hospice.

Life, what a precious but nebulous concept.

We were packed up and moved to the comfort care wing of the facility and the change was immediately apparent. There were no more late night and early morning awakenings for vital signs. The daily 4:30 a.m. blood draws stopped, Uncle Emil was no longer carted off to the dialysis treatment chair and there was an end to the anticipation and dread of another round of chemotherapy and its devastating side effects. Not surprisingly, he began to look better, he was more rested and although very weak was able to sit on the side of the bed for the first time in over two weeks.

The social worker, a part of the palliative care team arrived one morning and asked, "What are your plans for the future? We only keep patients here on this unit for a week to stabilize them and then will send them home with hospice support, or if that isn't available to a nursing home with hospice following."

Bradley C. Buckhout, M.D.

Uncle Emil had no home in Arizona. I was living in a rented room over the garage at the house that I own because the home was leased. He was not keen on a nursing home and in any case wasn't sure how he would pay for the expense of that care. The social worker then offered the hospice unit at the VA as a solution.

"Since you are a veteran, the VA will welcome you to their hospice unit. They don't have a time limit on the length of stay and I think with your diagnosis you will qualify for their care."

In short order we made our final move. The CLC (community living center) hospice unit of the VA did indeed welcome us. We were ushered in to a private room with a window overlooking a green lawn with trees. At the end of the hallway it was quiet so Emil could rest, but not on that first day. He was introduced to a confusing number of hospice team members all intent on making him comfortable and learning from him what they could provide to help him achieve his goals. He was seen by his bedside RN, a case manager, dietician, recreation therapist, nurse practitioner and his new physician with a group of students in tow. Each of these care givers had a well defined role and it was clear that they had functioned as a coordinated team for some time. Over the next few days, the social worker, chaplain and medical psychologist all made appearances and offered their services as needs came up.

The first afternoon, Dr. B sat down on the foot of the bed and began a conversation with Uncle Emil that first assessed his understanding of what was happening to him, what he had been told about his options and some sense of what his prognosis might be. I was there and was able to fill in some of the details that I had observed early in the course of the treatments when Uncle Emil was so sick that he had no recollection of what had happened. We then explored the meaning of hospice and discussed that the VA philosophy differs from most private hospice organizations by allowing concurrent care with oncologic services, treatment for other coexisting conditions and interventions for acute problems that might cause further discomfort or distress. That was very reassuring and left the door open for continuation of dialysis or perhaps even another round of chemo. It had now been long enough since the induction chemotherapy that the ill effects from the treatment were waning and Uncle Emil was regaining some desire to resume eating. Laying in bed waiting to die was not sounding as attractive as it once had. He thought that he had enough strength to perhaps be able to walk to the bathroom if he had a walker and some help.

Author's Note: Emil's position is not unique and there are times in severe illnesses when symptoms abate (often after curative attempts cease) and the patient begins to feel better. The specter of imminent demise begins to fade and the desire to continue living returns because the quality of life is worthy of continuation. This feeling of reprieve or escape from the hand of death is uplifting, encouraging and frequently leads to a rallying of spirit that buoys the patient and family but may cause everyone to begin to question the direction they have taken.

To get a better picture of where Emil was now in the continuum of his various problems lab work was obtained. His white count stood at 1500 meaning he was still at increased risk for infections. He was anemic and his platelet count was low enough that bleeding with little provocation could occur. Also worrisome was evidence that his kidneys were functioning very poorly. His creatinine, a waste product of protein metabolism normally excreted by the kidneys stood at 11.3, ten times the normal upper limit.

With this new information, the doctor returned and another discussion concerning goals of care ping-ponged back and forth:
1. Comfort care only with some physical therapy and the hope that he could get strong enough to walk to the bathroom.
2. Resume dialysis and physical therapy with the hope of going to the dining room for meals and to be able go outside again and enjoy the fresh air.
3. The most aggressive plan, attempt another chemotherapy cycle and hope that it wouldn't be as bad as it was the first time.

The horizon was unclear, the future unknown, but most assuredly less bright than it had been before all of this began. He called me and we talked at length, trying to make sense of what had happened and what was to come. He felt confused and uncertain but no longer had a feeling of helplessness. He had been given control of his options and was confident that the hospice team was working with him to improve his quality of life. We decided that evening that he would continue dialysis and would work with therapy to try to regain some of the strength that had melted away during his hospitalization.

I think we were all amazed at the progress he made over the next couple of weeks. He was able to get out of bed himself and walk to the bathroom and for short trips in the hall. His appetite improved and he went to the dining hall for the meals and camaraderie of the other veterans. With resumption of dialysis, his creatinine dropped to a tolerable level but his white cell count began an ominous ascension; 8000, 15,000, 23,000, 34,000 while his platelets headed down further 47,000, 31,000, 23,000 and he became anemic enough that he was dizzy sitting up and nearly fell getting out of bed. He received a transfusion of two units of red blood cells and these symptoms improved.

Dr. B returned and the subject of another round of chemotherapy was discussed. He had already spoken with the oncology service at the VA and it was their opinion that Emil would not be able to tolerate the ravages of another infusion cycle and that the likelihood of a favorable response was vanishingly small, they counseled against this plan of treatment.

It was not long after the decision had been made to allow the malignancy in the blood to run its natural course that Uncle Emil's condition began to change. He started to show evidence of small hemorrhages under the skin of his legs and abdomen. The doctor called these petechiae and were a result of his very low platelet count. These spots were a harbinger of something worse that would soon present itself. One morning Uncle Emil awoke with paralysis of the right side of his face and some difficulty lifting his right arm.

Dr B. examined him with his students hovering nearby. Uncle Emil, despite evidence that he was beginning to deteriorate again, returned to his performing persona and began his stand-up routine from a supine position this time. His recall of his old off-color jokes from as far back as twenty years ago was a little flawed but before long the five us were laughing after we provided explanations to the students, who were too young to understand some of the references. Dr. B snickered, "Emil, stop you're killing me!"

"Well, one of us anyway," came the retort from the horizontal stand-up comic.

The doctor explained that the combination of blood abnormalities had likely caused a small stroke and that there really were no good options for preventing further episodes or extension of the damage that had begun.

Bradley C. Buckhout, M.D.

"Perhaps it's time to reconsider whether we should continue dialysis. I think now we are just prolonging the inevitable and I am afraid that your ability to function is going to continue to decline. Is there anything that you need to do? Any tasks that you need to complete? Any people that you need to say goodbye to?" asked the doctor.

"My life has been full, I don't have any unresolved issues, these last couple of weeks have been a gift but I am at peace and whatever happens is OK with me. In ballpark terms, how long do you think this is going to take?" he calmly asked.

"I would think that without dialysis you are in the last weeks of this journey but I can't give you a guarantee. We will do what we can to make the last days as pain free, anxiety free and pleasant as we can," the doctor reassured. "Most patients with renal failure get progressively sleepier and one day just don't wake up."

"Thank you for that reassurance. I didn't know what to expect and that helps ease my mind. I don't want to linger with no hope of ever getting better."

Dialysis was discontinued and the large IV line was removed from his neck. His legs began to swell and elevating them didn't help much. The small skin hemorrhages proliferated and his right arm became more useless and finally the right leg stopped moving. Our conversations together became shorter as he would nod off after only a few minutes. We reminisced fondly about our shared history and then one evening while I was sitting at his bedside he simply stopped breathing.

I will miss Uncle Emil. His passing made me realize how uncertain our life is and that we need to make sure that we are living each day to the fullest and enjoying the time we are given. It also

When Caring Trumps Curing

made me consider my own inevitable mortality and that I need to consider the questions that Emil faced, sooner rather than later. I also have a different perspective on the role of palliative and hospice care in that they both work to improve the quality of life at the end and are not the "death panel" that some people envision them to be.

From the perspective of the palliative care physician, Emil's case offers several helpful lessons to consider. Americans have become much more mobile and families have scattered across the country. It can be difficult sometimes to maintain contact and having conversations about end of life planning does not easily fit into tweets, apparently the way people communicate today. Emil was fortunate to have a trusted family member on whom he could rely, but as you consider your situation you may want to cultivate friends in your locality if you have become distant from your relatives or you may want to pick up the phone and reconnect. It is wiser still to formally document your goals and wishes and to obtain agreement from the person who you would want to be your surrogate decision maker should your communication ability fail. Having this discussion and gaining agreement among family members now may prevent destruction of the remaining family ties when disagreements about care come up at a critical future time.

During the course of an ultimately terminal illness there is rarely a steady downhill rush. It is much more common to have a decline followed by a plateau and then a rally followed by further decline, another plateau and another rally until the end finally comes. These periods of rallying are difficult emotionally for the family and sometimes for the patient as well. Most patients however perceive that the body is dying and some parts are no longer serving their function with the same alacrity as before. It is not surprising to them therefore that the decline is continuing despite

Bradley C. Buckhout, M.D.

an occasional pause. Families on the other hand begin to question the decisions they have made to stop active treatment and to convert to an emphasis on comfort and not prolonging life. If we had only gotten another opinion, tried another round of chemotherapy, put in the feeding tube, etc., etc., he would still be alive. These laments are heard frequently and can be a great source of guilt and dissatisfaction if not dealt with early in the process of discussions with the patient and care team. Clarity in expectations and prognosis are the greatest antidote but as in this case, these are sometimes difficult for doctors to provide. Being present for family conferences with the care team and having questions ready is your best tool but recognizing the uncertainty with which this information can be provided will help to reassure. Remember, milk has an expiration date, patients don't.

Chapter 6
LYNN

I hadn't spoken with my sister since she left Salt Lake City with that worthless Greg eighteen years ago. She met him during her stint in the Navy and perhaps that common experience is what bonded them together initially. I guess I was a bit too vocal in my opinions about him and his drinking and didn't consider that there must have been something that she saw that I couldn't. I know that I had hurt her feelings badly and she swore that she would never speak to me again but life has a strange way of bringing the family back together again.

I was shocked to hear from her when she called in July of 2015. But even after not hearing from her for so long I could tell by the quiver in her voice that she was scared. I will recount what she told me to fill in the story of how we reconnected. When they left, she and Greg had moved to a little community near Lake Quinault on the Olympic peninsula in Washington and he had gotten a job with a forestry company. Lynn was busy with her art work and was inspired by the beauty of the lake and forest. They had a son, a nephew I unfortunately did not get to meet until he was much older. Things were going well, for a while.

Then Greg was injured at work, was hospitalized and then confined to bed. He began to drink, heavily. Finances became strained and he became anxious, irritable and withdrawn, his PTSD flared and their relationship deteriorated and finally broke.

Bradley C. Buckhout, M.D.

Lynn was left alone with her son Darren, without steady income in an isolated little town in the woods. She was eventually desperate enough to send her son to live with our brother and his wife and children in Seattle. She stayed in the cabin and worked at the little gift shop at the Lodge and slipped into a deep depression. I believe that was the reason she didn't seek medical attention when she first noticed the tenderness and then the lump in her right breast. She wasn't taking care of herself and was eating to relieve her distress so her weight climbed to a very unhealthy 236 pounds. The weight gain may have hidden the increasing size of the mass in her breast for a time but eventually the skin started to redden and then dimple over the tumor. Finally, in 2015 while on a trip to Seattle to visit Darren and our brother's family a spot of blood began to expand slowly on her blouse. Alarmed, her sister-in-law took her to the bathroom and what they discovered frightened both of them. There was an angry looking bleeding ulceration of the skin of her breast.

With much cajoling her brother and sister-in-law were able to get her to go to an emergency room in Seattle. She was admitted to the VA hospital and was seen by a surgeon and then an oncologist. It was plainly evident that she had an advanced cancer of the breast. Studies were completed to evaluate the extent of the disease and it was discovered that the cancer had already spread to her brain. Her prognosis was not good. She was told that she likely had 3 months to live. Radiation and chemotherapy could be started but they were unlikely to extend her life more than a few months at best and might make her ill and fatigued. Surgery could be done to remove the affected breast so that she would not have an open wound, but it would not change her prognosis.

Lynn deliberated, took stock of her life and elected to not pursue any of those options but instead selected the support of the hospital's palliative care team. Darren was now eighteen and had enlisted in the Air Force and would be leaving for boot camp. She felt that he was going to the military and would be shepherded into manhood in the rigid structure provided there. She was becoming weaker, her appetite had decreased and she was having headaches, pain in her chest wall and was needing wound care on a daily basis. She was admitted to a CLC in Spokane in June of 2015.

She had been in the facility with hospice support for about a month when she called me. She was scared, as I mentioned, but was also outwardly calm and apparently at peace with her decision to not receive palliative chemo or radiation. She had requested that care be focused on preserving her comfort for the few months she had remaining. We spoke for a time and I offered to come and see her. Initially she thanked me but asked me not to come. I agreed, but offered to come whenever she felt that she needed me. We talked periodically and she never asked me to visit but on one call it was clear that something had changed. She kept losing her train of thought and her words sounded slurred. When I got off the phone with Lynn, I called our brother and he said, "If you want to see your sister you better go now, she has lost a lot of weight and they think the brain metastases are growing".

I hopped in the car and drove the 9 1/2 hours to Spokane to be with her by the next morning. I honestly didn't recognize her. She had changed her hair color, she was heavier than I remembered and her smile was a little crooked, but her face lit up when she saw me and after a long embrace the tears started to flow. "I'm so sorry,..." was all she could get out between the sobs.

"Me too, what can I do to help? I can't let you go through this alone." Through that whole day, interrupted by her naps, we reminisced and brought each other up to date on our lives. If you have been close to someone, you have experienced the feeling that no time has elapsed in your relationship even if many years have gone by since you last sat together. That was how this reunion went, we were sisters once again, once inseparable; separated and now rejoined.

She was comfortable in the VA and was being well taken care of, a role that I was not sure that I could replicate at the time and so I left her there after a week and returned home. We spoke often and she surprisingly, did much better than any of her doctors expected. She was alive at three months, five months, nine months, ten months after the diagnosis when she had been told by her oncologist, "You have an incurable intraductal carcinoma of the breast. It has already spread to your brain. Our best guess is that you have perhaps three months to live." The lesson here is that prognostication is an inexact art. There are many indicators that can be used to assist a clinician in predicting when a patient may pass away but the truth is that these can only be used to "ballpark" a time period that one might be expected to finally succumb. For example, someone with heart disease, copd and diabetes who required hospitalization in the last year could reasonably be expected to die in the next few years. A patient with metastatic lung cancer would likely survive many months to a year. A seventy year old man with prostate cancer that has spread to the bones with a rising serum calcium may reasonably expect weeks to months. If that same patient's condition has progressed further so he is bed bound and not eating well, his time can likely be measured in days to weeks.

For patients, no matter what the underlying illness, who are no longer eating or drinking and who are difficult to arouse and engage in conversation, hours to a few days is the likely timeline. When the normal rhythmic breathing pattern is no longer

When Caring Trumps Curing

operating and mottling of the extremities is evident, the body is in its final hours. As the end approaches there are common signs as the body begins to shut down that are recognizable making the prognostication more accurate the nearer death looms.

One of the strongest predictive scales, originally created for oncology patients is a measure of function. Known as the ECOG scale (for Eastern Cooperative Oncology Group). The numeric scale starts at 0 for patients who have disease but no physical symptoms and increases as the disease process consumes the patient's vitality.

1 = Able to carry on normal activity but not physically strenuous tasks
2 = Able to do self care tasks but not able to perform work, up & about >50% of the day
3 = In bed or chair >50% needs assistance with self care
4 = Totally dependent on others for care, bed bound
5 = Deceased

Even the medically untrained can make a fairly accurate prognostication using this evaluation. Who do you think will live longer; a woman with metastatic colon cancer who is still able to putter about in her garden or the woman with a similar cancer who has to be ceiling lifted to her wheelchair due to the loss of strength in her legs? If you chose the first woman, you have a feel for the concept. I find this applicable to all chronic illnesses and find it helpful in explaining to patients where they may be in their disease trajectory. It is much more readily apparent than the meaning of some lab tests or scan results and can give people a tangible, easily demonstrable measure of "Doc, how am I doing?"

Over the many months she was in Spokane, her breast wound began to become more painful and so the doses of morphine increased progressively. She was not sleeping well at night and so another medication was added for sleep and an antidepressant was added to try to elevate her mood. When we talked in May, it was apparent that something was wrong. Lynn was not herself, she sounded very down, like she was giving up. She was having trouble keeping up with our conversation and didn't laugh at my attempts at humor like she usually would.

"Lynn, I'm coming to get you. This is too hard to be apart and you having to go through this by yourself. Mia wants to be with you too."

She offered only token resistance to my offer for her to come and move in with us. My eleven year old daughter rode with me the following weekend to pick her up in our minivan and to bring her back to Salt Lake. We contacted the local VA and they helped us with referrals to a local hospice agency. Soon after Lynn arrived, we converted our den downstairs to her hospice lair, complete with an electric hospital bed, posters of the Washington forest, a lava lamp, Native American dream catchers and pottery. Our family bonded more closely and I would find Mia at her bedside drawing or writing stories with her. Lynn ate little, sipping on a can of Ensure that she would nurse through an entire day. Due to her wound and the smell that necrotic tissue and old blood produce she showered every day. This began to pose a problem because our shower is on the second floor and Lynn was becoming weak enough the we had to put a chair on the landing of the stairway to give her a place to sit and rest so she could make it all the way to the second floor. She became short of breath from showering and then one day she fell coming back down the stairs.

This frightened all of us and my husband began to hang on to her with each trip up and down for her daily shower. She still fell twice more when her legs gave out. Even though she had lost ninety pounds during the last year she was still not a frail small woman and my husband could not hold her up. Thankfully, other than some impressive bruising of her right leg and hip she was not injured but it was becoming clear that we were getting to a point that soon we were going to need more help.

As it turned out, the stars began to align. Lynn's son, Darren had recently been transferred to Luke Air Force Base in Phoenix. The Salt Lake VA social worker contacted the Phoenix VA CLC and requested that Lynn be allowed to transfer there so that she could be closer to her son who coincidentally had just been discovered to have a mass in his right thigh that needed to be removed. Lynn was accepted and we packed up the minivan and headed for the sunny Southwest for the Christmas Holiday... Lynn's last.

The room we were given was on the first floor with a view of a patio garden and after settling Lynn into bed Mia and I made the room her home. The posters from her room, her lava lamp and bean bag chair and rug on the floor. Incense and music with the subdued lighting almost made our visitors believe we weren't in a nursing home hospice room. The staff was welcoming and accommodating and wanted to make this transition as easy as possible. Mia, wearing her reindeer antlers, greeted each new visitor of the medical team that came to evaluate and assist Lynn.

When the CLC hospice team first met Lynn, her sister Tina and Mia, the first impression was of the warmth and caring that Lynn had received for the many months at Tina's home. Her diagnosis had been made sixteen months ago and although she was having some word finding difficulty and her speech was soft and slow she was awake and alert and able to communicate her needs. She had been having difficulty with making decisions and was needing help with her adls (activities of daily living) at the time she

Bradley C. Buckhout, M.D.

transferred to us. She was still able to get up from her bed and walk slowly to the bathroom in her room. Our shower room is down the hall and when she arrived she was able to walk there with her sister assisting for balance.

Her right arm was her major physical concern as it felt "dead" with painful pins and needles and numbness and swelling. She had been on gabapentin in the past but had been discontinued by the hospice for some reason and since it was felt to have been helpful before, we elected to resume it at a conservative dose. The other issue was the wound on the right breast which was increasing in size and was bleeding, with some persistence that was on occasion difficult to stop. Dressing changes were required daily and she still showered every day to try to reduce the odor from the tissue that was dying and sloughing as the cancer cells outstripped their blood supply. Lynn had made it clear that she had accepted the terminal nature of her disease and she was very grateful that she had been given nearly two years longer than her initial prognosis to share with her sister and her dear niece.

What determines the final steps leading ultimately to death? The physiologic, metabolic, anatomic changes can all be relatively well defined and are seen with reasonable predictability. What remains an uncertainty is the nature of the catalyst that begins the inexorable cascade of events that lead to the final silence. Is there a final resolution of a problem that has plagued the patient, a relationship repaired, a wish fulfilled, a dream achieved? Sometimes there appears to be nothing left to live for, the quality of life has dwindled to the point that the end is a beloved release from the torments of the body. It is on rare occasions that the final necessary act has been explicitly expressed in advance, such as, "when my daughter gets here and says her goodbyes it will be my time". Mostly the time is personal and known to only the patient. I am not convinced that we have control over the precise time of our death but there are many patients in whom it is apparent that the will to live has finally departed.

The signs that the time is approaching are probably more signs that the complex interactions of the multiple systems that make up our miraculous bodies are beginning to fail. But from some perspectives the same signs can be interpreted as the patient has given up, has lost the will to live, is too tired to go on. Sleeping more, not wanting to get out of bed, loss of appetite, slowing of thought processes, decreasing urine output, slowing of respirations, stagnation of blood with cooling and mottling of the skin are all evidence that the end is near in any number of chronic illnesses.

Lynn apparently had much to do, relationships to mend, to see her son again and to perhaps even see the birth of his wife's first baby. Her faith was strong and she had no fear about what was coming next. She actually viewed her disease as having a silver lining. It had rekindled the love between sisters and brought Mia into her life. While under our care, she had many conversations with the chaplain and shared her happiness to be finally going 'home' (to Heaven) when she died. There had been many changes that the cancer had caused, that had been painful, but it also had caused dramatic changes in her vision of who she was as a woman.

She had enough strength to go to her daughter-in-law's baby shower but she was extremely fatigued by the effort that this took and she spent the next days in bed, mostly asleep. One day Lynn discovered some new lumps at the base of her neck. Perhaps she had slept with her head in an awkward position she thought, but the knots were still there the next morning.

Bradley C. Buckhout, M.D.

The doctor came in that afternoon with the wound nurse practitioner to check on the results of the new dressing that was being used for her breast wound. It was apparently helping as the dressing had not become saturated with blood since it was applied the day before.

"Hey Doc, there is something wrong with the side of my neck. I found some bumps a couple of days ago. Could you take a look?"

"Sure Lynn, let me check them out. Is there anything else you've noticed, any pain, sore throat, difficulty swallowing?"

"No, just the lumps."

As the doctor examined her he spoke to the NP with him. "The swelling in the arm hasn't increased and there is no redness. At the base of the neck there is a cluster of hard nodes that feel matted together deep to the subq tissues." He looked at me and then to Lynn and said, "I am afraid that these are lymph nodes and that the cancer has spread to them, that's why you can feel them now."

"So the cancer is spreading? That sucks"! Lynn sighed.

The doctor reminded her that this was not the first evidence the cancer had spread and as a matter of fact the reason she had not elected therapy back when her breast cancer was diagnosed was that it already spread to her brain. He then reviewed her medications and she assured him that she was not having significant pain and that nothing needed to be changed.

"Since the cancer cells are growing here they are likely growing elsewhere, I would like to add some dexamethasone to try to prevent swelling in your brain which could cause seizures or symptoms like you've had a stroke."

"The last time I was on steroids I felt like I wanted to kill somebody," Lynn replied. We all agreed that would not be good for anyone and it was decided to stay the course for now.

Mia and I had to return to Salt Lake for two weeks and Darren, who was off work following the surgery on his thigh, was able to come and spend time with his mom. When we got back, she was more peaceful and the two of them had been able to share their wishes and hopes. She was encouraged that he was going to be a happy successful young man and a good father when his son arrived.

Lynn had now been in the hospice in Phoenix for fifty days. In the short time we were away there had developed evidence of further disease progression. She was nauseated frequently, even the meager amount of fluid intake that she had been taking was no longer tolerated. She was having difficulty taking medications and the medical team was concerned that without IV access they would not be able to manage her pain and the increasing air hunger that she was feeling. The other concern was the effects of suddenly stopping the opioids that she had been on for so long. Withdrawal would be very unpleasant and an unnecessary additional burden for her to bear. Lynn initially resisted the placement of an IV line believing that receiving fluids would prolong her life, something she repeatedly stressed that she did not want. The doctor returned to check on her and discuss her decision and his concerns.

"Lynn, I know you are starting to have trouble swallowing but there are some medications that you need to help keep you comfortable."

Bradley C. Buckhout, M.D.

"But doctor, I don't want this to last any longer than it absolutely has to, I am ready to go," she stated calmly.

"We are not giving you anything that is going to change how long you are going to live. But we don't want whatever time you have left to be filled with pain or nausea and the anxiety that feeling short of breath will cause."

"Thank you, that helps, I guess you can have the nurse put the IV in, if there are still places that will work after all this time."

After the line was started, they began a hydromorphone drip and you could see Lynn relax. She was actually able to get some rest. She had no appetite and only took sips of juice to keep her mouth moist.

Mia and I were sleeping in her room, Mia in her beanbag chair and me on the other unoccupied bed in the room. During the day there was staff in and out of her room many times each hour. She was able to receive additional doses of hydromorphone when the pain in her back or chest got bad. She found that it also helped relieve the feeling that she wasn't getting enough air. At night unfortunately there are fewer staff and I would sometimes have to wander the hall to find someone to come and help. Being with someone you love and watching them suffer is the hardest thing I have ever had to do. It was one of the reasons I was not disappointed when Lynn suggested coming to Phoenix to the VA to be closer to her son. We had mended all of the bad feelings and intentional and unintentional slights that had kept us apart for years and honestly I was feeling like we needed more help than what the home hospice caregivers in Salt Lake could offer.

The hospice providers here were more numerous, there was someone around constantly. The chaplain was very helpful and sat with Lynn to share scripture and hymns. Recreation therapy had a big selection of soothing music that we had playing on the CD player when we weren't talking. The medical team did what could be done for the smell from the flesh that was dying in her breast and they were able to stop the bleeding from the raw tissue. They monitored her pain levels and the amount of extra doses she needed and adjusted the rate of her drip until the need for boluses decreased. Her breathing continued to be a struggle and although they didn't take an x-ray the nurse practitioner was able to tell by listening that her right lung was being compressed by fluid filling the chest cavity.

Cancer cells cause inflammation and when on the pleural surface, fluid in large quantities can be produced. The fluid will fill the space between the chest wall and the lung, compressing it so the small air sacs (alveoli) collapse. They can then no longer oxygenate the blood or expel the carbon dioxide. Observing at the bedside, an increase in respiratory rate will be noticeable, often with shallow quick breaths. Supplemental oxygen is frequently offered and may be helpful in providing oxygen to the alveoli that are still open and functioning. This may give some relief of the sense of air hunger and shortness of breath. The plastic nasal prongs however can be irritating and patients, particularly if they are suffering from delirium, will pull them off. When more oxygen is needed, oxygen masks can be offered but there is often a paradoxic sense of smothering with these and they are not well tolerated. These devices are being used to provide comfort at the end of life. If they are not, especially if they are a source of irritation, they can be dispensed with rather than restraining the patient to enforce their use. In most situations, medications, particularly opiates or anti-anxiety medications, are more effective for patient comfort.

Bradley C. Buckhout, M.D.

Lynn began the final decline to her goal the morning after Valentine's Day. She was flushed and hot to touch, sleeping and not easy to arouse. She would however, still squeeze my hand when I spoke to her. Research has suggested that hearing is the last sense to cease functioning and we encourage family members at the bedside to continue to speak with, pray with, sing to and reassure their loved one even after it appears they are no longer able to respond. She appeared to be comfortable, at peace and awaiting her last breath.

The doctor sat with me and said that Lynn likely had developed pneumonia from the atelectasis (the compressed alveoli). With her damaged immune system being fully engaged battling the cancer she would likely develop an overwhelming infection (sepsis) and even with antibiotics would not likely survive. He reasserted his assent with Lynn's wish to do nothing to prolong her dying process and I agreed without hesitation.

As the hours ticked past, Lynn began to have this disturbing wet sounding irregular breathing noise. It sounded like she was drowning in her own secretions. The nurses turned her to her side, swabbed her mouth and used a suction tip to clear the mucus from her mouth. That all helped for a while. She started to moan and they had to turn her to her back again as they couldn't roll her on her right side due to her wound and swollen arm. On her back, the gurgling started again, what is frequently called the "death rattle". I don't think Lynn was aware of it but for Mia and me and Darren we all just wanted it to stop, one way or another...

In addition to the concern that we all had that this noise was an indication that she was struggling to breathe, it also accentuated the fact that her breathing was no longer the regular in and out that we all take for granted. There were long pauses 2...3...4...

seconds with no breath. We were all holding our breaths unconsciously...is it over? Was that the last breath? Is Lynn finally home? and then she would resume, rapid deep breaths that would then become slower and more shallow and then pause again 3...4....5... seconds. Gurgle...rasp...pause. The evening nurse came in and gave her an injection of something called robinul and the horrible wet rasping almost went away.

The nurse came back to check on us at 10:00pm. We had all dozed off, me on the bed, Darren in the recliner and Mia dozing in the chair next to the bed holding Lynn's hand. Lynn's face was pale. No longer flushed, her lips were a faint bluish color and she was no longer breathing. Her journey was finally completed. The tears flowed. Tears of loss but also tears of relief, Lynn was no longer suffering. For me, I had my sister back if only for a short time. Mia was able to meet her aunt and to learn life lessons of faith and courage. Darren reconnected with his mother. Her strength in dealing with the adversity she faced will hopefully inspire him to find the strength he needs to confront his medical issues as he builds his new family.

Bradley C. Buckhout, M.D.

Chapter 7
TAMI

I had been working at the VA for just over three years, caring for primarily aging male veterans whose loss of ability to function independently had necessitated their admission to our nursing home. The vast majority of veterans of our previous wars were male so it stands to reason that elderly males would dominate our population of residents. It is with that background that we admitted Tami, a unique veteran, to the CLC. She had been in the Air Force, serving in a non-combat role stateside before medical issues forced her retirement. As a teenager, she was plagued with headaches, fairly typical of migraines with hormonal cycling fluctuations in frequency and intensity. She was able to gain sufficient control of her pain to enlist but during her service new symptoms began to appear.

She had transient vision loss and double vision prior to the onset of some of her hemi-cranial pounding headaches. Initially these were interpreted as a migraine aura, a not uncommon phenomenon. Alterations of her migraine medications were tried but the vision impairment became more persistent even without the subsequent head pain. Her neurologist, concerned that there was something new causing this problem drew labs and requested an MRI of the brain. The images revealed the white matter plaques typical of multiple sclerosis. This neurodegenerative disease presents most commonly in young females and has a variable course of progression. The neurologic deficits it causes are extremely variable between individuals. Response to therapies can be unpredictable and there is unfortunately, a tendency to progressive loss of function, usually over many years.

When Caring Trumps Curing

Tami was seen by internationally respected multiple sclerosis experts and she received the most advanced care that was available at the time. As is typical of the disease, there were periods of progression when new symptoms would appear and further loss of function would become apparent. These episodes would be followed by variable intervals of stability when her losses would plateau. One unfortunate constant however, was her headaches... She was tried on each new product as it became available, she was given every type of preventative and abortive medication on the market, a total of twenty-six different products according to a medication review that was completed when she was admitted to our unit. It was during this review that we discovered that she had been receiving intravenous meperidine (demerol) on a regular basis in the emergency room to obtain relief from her debilitating headache episodes. We were even more surprised to find that due to her poor peripheral veins a port for intravenous access had been implanted under the skin of her chest.

What had happened to this unfortunate thirty year old female veteran that necessitated her admission to our nursing home? She had been receiving care at home from her family with the help of visiting nurses but the dynamics there had changed recently. Her brother had been called to active duty and had left for a military base in Germany. Her father had just gone, apparently not able to emotionally deal with his daughter's illness. Her mother had to return to work for at least eight hours each day to support them. Tami was no longer able to walk and had been confined to her manual wheelchair. The damage to her nervous system caused severe spasticity of her extremities, she was not able to control her hands well enough to be able to feed herself or hold a cup for drinking. So, while her mom was working, Tami had no access to food or water and her weight had declined steadily.

Bradley C. Buckhout, M.D.

The nurses and social workers visiting the home were concerned and with mom they tried to provide care that would support them so that Tami could remain in her mother's home. Adequate caregiver time in the home was difficult to achieve and Tami was visibly losing ground. She was fearful of being alone and her mother could not be with her long enough each day to provide the care she needed. The eventual painful discussion concerning placement in a facility was received with angry resistance from both Tami and her mother and by feelings of guilt and abandonment despite its clear necessity. Finally, on another trip to the emergency room for one of her headaches, it was discovered that there were more serious issues. She also had a urinary infection and her weight had reached 88 pounds, down from her normal of 132. It was then that they accepted the fact, Tami needed round the clock care.

I will never forget the conversation I had with Tami the day I met her. She was alone in her room seated in her manual wheelchair, her arms in constant rhythmic, uncontrollable motion and her legs twitching unrelentingly at a different frequency. She had a mild bobbing motion of her head and her eyes behind her glasses appeared to have difficulty fixing on me as we spoke. She was unnaturally thin, bringing to mind the British model from the 60's, Twiggy.

"So, what do you understand about the reason you're here?" I asked her during our introduction.

"I guess I've come here to die," was her somewhat unsettling and blunt but likely realistic response.

"Do you think this is the place that you want to be? You are the only female on the unit and you are three or four decades younger than the rest of the patients." I counseled. With a lopsided grin that we have all come to recognize prior to one of Tami's off the wall comments she replied, "I figured as much but it's OK...I like the Old Foxes".

Our first order of business was to learn about Tami's view of her existence and to what extent she wanted us to do things to keep her alive. This is termed the goals of care discussion. Sometimes, the goals and desires are very clear and there are no conflicts to be resolved. In Tami's case, her goals were clear and this conversation was completed easily. Tami clearly was competent to make decisions concerning her care. Her mother however, was intimately involved in her care and her life. It was therefore important that she was aware of Tami's wishes and concerns so that we were all on the same page moving forward.

Tami was definite and resolute. She is planning to outlive her mother. She therefore wants everything done to keep her alive. She wishes cardiac resuscitation and to be placed on a ventilator to assist her breathing if that became necessary. These were certainly not unreasonable wishes for someone in their third decade of life but perhaps less so knowing what lies ahead for people suffering with multiple sclerosis.

Our second priority was to deal with her severe weight loss from lack of nutrition. At the time of admission, her swallowing reflex was already becoming unreliable and there was a significant risk that she could aspirate food or liquids into her trachea or even bronchi were we to try to replenish her wasted body strictly by the oral route. Tami and her mother both agreed that placement of a feeding tube, although not without some risks, would be the most expedient method of repletion.

If the reader doesn't mind, I would like to digress for a moment concerning the issue of feeding tubes. There are often misconcep-

Bradley C. Buckhout, M.D.

tions about these devices, the reasons for their use, the risks and benefits associated with them that can lead to contentious discussions between family members, patients and their medical providers.

There are two basic types of feeding tubes. One can be inserted at the bedside and is referred to as a nasogastric tube (NG tube). This is traditionally done as a temporary bridge technique in adults but nasogastric feedings in infants are often utilized for longer term support. The NG tube is also used as a suction device, to empty the stomach of its contents in a variety of situations. This type of tube can be advanced into the duodenum or even the jejunum for feedings which is particularly helpful if there are stomach emptying problems. By placing the feedings further down in the small bowel the risk of aspirating the tube feedings is diminished although not completely eliminated.

A more advanced form of the naso-jejunal tube is called a Duo-tube and it is placed using an endoscope by a gastroenterologist or by an interventional radiologist through the nose and into the second portion of the small intestine. It is actually two tubes in one with the first, a larger lumen that stops in the stomach allowing it to be decompressed or medications to be delivered and the finer tube which passes through the first, terminating in the small intestine where nutrition and water are delivered.

The second type of feeding tube requires a surgical procedure performed most commonly by a gastroenterologist or interventional radiologist and in some situations by a general surgeon at the end of an abdominal procedure. These are known as PEG tubes, G tubes, G-J tubes. The designation refers to the fact that the entry point of the tube into the digestive tract is the stomach (gastric) through a puncture wound made through the wall of the abdomen. PEG refers to a percutaneous endoscopic gastrostomy tube. This tube is placed using an endoscope passed from above down the esophagus into the stomach. The lighted end of the scope is then turned up towards the abdominal wall and a large needle is passed through the skin, fat and muscle and through the wall of the stomach at the location of the light. A wire is then passed through the needle and is grasped by a forceps protruding from the scope. From this point the gastrostomy tube is placed either by pushing it directly through the abdominal wall or is pulled down the esophagus after being attached to the wire near the mouth and pulled out from within the stomach.

There is also a technique done by interventional radiologists without the endoscope using x-ray imaging to locate the stomach and point of insertion. As I frequently tell patients there is always something that we as physicians can do to you but I'm not so certain that it is always for you. A feeding tube for Tami was an appropriate intervention, without it her goal of outliving her mother was not going to happen.

Although insertion problems are rare, bleeding, stomach contents leaking into the abdomen, perforation of another organ, infection of the insertion site can happen. The most common and concerning complication seen is aspiration of the gastric contents or tube feeding fluid into the lungs leading to pneumonitis. This issue alone has lead to the significant controversy concerning placement of feeding tubes in the debilitated elderly. Commonly found in nursing homes after a stroke or with dementia which prevents normal swallowing, these frail elderly often have a feeding tube that was placed in the acute care hospital. At the time the tube was contemplated the family was likely convinced that it was the right thing to do to keep their loved one alive. It was not likely explained that the aspiration pneumonia associated with these devices is actually one of the most common causes of death in this population. It is interesting to view information that

Bradley C. Buckhout, M.D.

has been collected nationally to see huge variations in the use of feeding tubes in the nursing home population. The medical care from state to state does not vary that significantly. Apparently, the philosophy of care for the elderly, or if one wishes to be more cynical, the rate of reimbursement for the procedure and care after placement of the tubes does. The data from 2006 showed that the lowest utilization of feeding tubes in elderly residents of nursing homes was in Nebraska at 3.8%. The highest use occurred in the District of Columbia at an incredible rate of 44.8%!

The rate of aspiration pneumonia in tube-fed patients ranges from approximately 5% to 58% depending on the factors of the patient noted below and also the vigilance of the care center staff where the feedings are being administered. Aspiration unfortunately can occur without obvious evidence of vomiting or regurgitation and is recognized by the development of signs of respiratory distress or pneumonia. Nasoenteral (beyond the stomach) and gastrostomy tubes are felt by some to prevent aspiration, although evidence is lacking to support this belief.

Additional risk factors for the development of aspiration pneumonia include advanced age, the presence of esophagitis on endoscopy and/or a history of gastroesophageal reflux. The risk is also increased if there have been prior episodes of aspiration or pneumonia. Impaired level of consciousness, neurologic deficits, poor oral hygiene or use of sedative medications also should be causes to consider carefully the use of a feeding tube. Although acid suppression may help with symptoms of reflux, it does not prevent aspiration pneumonia. Pro-motility drugs such as metoclopramide (reglan) may reduce the risk of aspiration in patients with evidence of delayed gastric emptying. Improving oral care in nursing home residents has demonstrated lowered risk of pneumonia in this fragile population. Tube feedings can also lead to abdominal bloating and diarrhea with resultant damage to the skin of the buttocks and potentially the development of sacral/buttock wounds. Modifications of the feeding formulas can be tried as can the method of delivery, from bolus to continuous feeds or vice versa. Occasionally, to control the excessive stooling, medications with their inherent side effects, are required. There are also frequent metabolic issues with electrolyte disturbances, blood sugar control may become difficult, over-hydration leading to low sodium occurs in as many as 25% of people receiving tube feedings.

The tubes themselves can cause significant complications when they are inadvertently inserted into the trachea, intracranially or perforate the esophagus or stomach. As many as 25% of inserted tubes are dislodged and require reinsertion with the inherent risks with each insertion. Taping them in place, hiding the tube under an abdominal binder can help preserve the tube but in a demented patient with all day to work at it, the tube is not likely going to remain in place without a very vigilant family or staff.

Tami's PEG tube was placed without complications by the GI department and the feedings were begun with an impressive and steady gain in her weight. Within five months she had regained her original weight and finally stabilized at 142 pounds. As a consequence of her severe weight loss, Tami had been amenorrheic for several years but with the return of her normal body weight her cycles resumed. One day I encountered her in the hall in her wheelchair with her knees tied together with a brightly colored scarf.

"Hey Tami, what's up with the scarf?" I inquired.

"Birth control," came her reply and she began to weep.

Bradley C. Buckhout, M.D.

When I expressed concern for why she was crying she touchingly replied, "I have parts I will never get to use. I will never have a child and now I'm being reminded every month".

To reduce her distress, we began depoprovera injections to decrease the frequency of her menses. This worked well. The next issue she had to face was, in part, related to her hormonal abnormalities. She began to complain of back pain, "The nurses broke my back," more specifically.

Tami could no longer stand or transfer from her bed to her chair but our facility is equipped with ceiling lifts that use a sling to move patients safely from place to place. The sling does flex the patient at the waist as they are lifted but there is really little trauma with the procedure. I initially did not take Tami seriously as she continued to behave in her usual unique fashion and did not seek an increase in the amount of pain medication that she was receiving. After she made the statement a second time, "The nurses broke my back again," a week later we sent her for x-rays of her lumbar spine. There was some osteoporosis reported but no fracture identified in her lumbar vertebrae. It wasn't until her pain complaints persisted that we got the real answer when we ordered a CT scan of her spine and discovered multiple compression fractures of her lumbar spine. In retrospect this made sense. Tami had been functionally post-menopausal due to her very low body weight and she had not done any weight bearing activity for years. Despite being on calcium and vitamin D supplements, her skeleton was also deteriorating. Since she could not take oral medications, we elected to begin her on a once yearly dose of zoledronic acid to protect her from further bone loss and to promote healing of her fractures.

In addition to her back pain, Tami had continuous headaches. It was sometimes difficult to tell how much she was suffering but she was relentless in her request for medications to free her of this affliction. After reviewing her list of medications again, I started back down the list. "Do you remember what happened when you took propranolol?"

"It didn't work."

"How about depakote?"

"If it helped I'd probably still be on it, right?"

We went through a dozen or so medications used for migraine prevention or relief and eventually circled back to her original request, IV demerol. This opiate has very limited use any longer and is a poor choice for chronic use due to active metabolites which can accumulate causing some significant side effects. Admittedly in Tami's case she seemed to tolerate the medication and appeared to slowly melt into her chair with the relaxation achieved with each injection. Not being happy with this option, I spoke with her neurologist who gave a very palliative care type of answer. "I agree that demerol is not a good long term option. But honestly with the quality of life she has, I'm OK with you ordering that medication, if it gives her a little relief or pleasure."

We continued with further attempts at replacement and adjunctive medications, relaxation techniques, guided imagery (this did not go well as the image used was of a dolphin playfully cutting through the waves...Tami apparently doesn't swim and is afraid of water). We offered hypnosis, acupuncture, massage and any number of distractions to little appreciable benefit. Our concern was Tami's requests for the demerol doses kept increasing in size and frequency and providers became uncomfortable justifying continuation of this drug. Ultimately, we converted her to a

Bradley C. Buckhout, M.D.

fentanyl patch. I'm not sure this achieved completely what she was desiring, but eventually her headache complaints decreased and she stopped asking for demerol.

Over the years on our unit, now approaching eleven, Tami has become the Queen of the CLC. Her 40th birthday was celebrated with a crown, floor length red robe, scepter and a throne built specially for her wheelchair. Her 'subjects' have an abiding affection for her perhaps in part due to her off color comments, her encyclopedic knowledge of famous American serial killers and her good nature despite the cruel fate she has been dealt.

Multiple sclerosis is a progressively debilitating condition that destroys the myelin insulation of the nervous system causing it to "short out" in any number of ways. The deterioration is extremely variable in how it attacks each patient. Another of our long term patients who has had MS for over 45 years is essentially a quadriplegic. Tami has no use of her legs but she can move her arms, albeit with uncoordinated ballistic jerking type motions. She claims to have no control over this but I have cautioned any male student accompanying me on rounds to stand at a safe distance with hands clasped in front to protect themselves from these "spasms".

Our other veteran retains the ability to swallow and handle his secretions and he can still be fed a normal diet. Tami on the other hand, has not been able to safely eat for over a decade. She also has trouble swallowing her own saliva and her speech frequently becomes wet and gurgly.

"Hey Tami, why are you talking like Nemo?" I tease.

"Shut up, Dork," she gurgles.

When Caring Trumps Curing

It is with sadness that we all have been a witness to her slow decline. In the past, comical exchanges with her were an enjoyable part of the day and now it is almost impossible to understand what she is saying. She has suffered several recent infections. Pneumonia developed due to her weak, impaired cough and a urinary tract infection after her failing nervous system lead to significant retention of urine. We have been able to successfully treat these infections and she has recovered but with each episode she is a little weaker and a little closer to the end of this long journey.

I have had many conversations with her mother during her decade with us about what she would want should Tami develop respiratory failure and require a ventilator to continue living. In the past, she could not come to grips with the concept that her daughter was dying. She would always defer making a decision, "until I speak to her brother and get his opinion…I'll get back to you." I would never hear from her until I called months later, with the same result.

It was not until this last year that she tearfully acknowledged the decline that we have all been trying to deny. Tami can no longer inhale when a cigarette is held to her lips, one of the few pleasures remaining to her. She has a big screen TV on the wall of her room but is showing little interest in the choice of movies so the nurses make selections for her.

"I know she is dying and there is nothing you can do to stop her disease. I just don't want my girl to suffer."

"We all agree and we don't want to have anything unnecessary done to Tami. I have spoken with her and she told me she doesn't want to be transferred to the intensive care unit to be put on a ventilator," I told Tami's mom.

Bradley C. Buckhout, M.D.

"She doesn't want to leave this unit where she knows everyone and she is treated like family. What I would request is that you talk with her and let her know that you are in agreement with her decision, as painful as that is for you to consider."

This difficult exchange is very common in the palliative care world for any number of chronic, slowly progressive debilitating conditions that don't suddenly take the sufferer. The course is often an indolent decline punctuated by an acute worsening of the situation when an infection intervenes or another stroke takes more of the brain out of commission. Multiple sclerosis, ALS (amyotrophic lateral sclerosis), dementia, strokes, heart failure, renal failure, cancer can all follow this course. Because of this reality, it is vitally important to begin to consider what the final acts of life will be and where they will be played out.

We had visited these questions earlier but repetition is frequently necessary to overcome the disbelief and resistance that family members have when they are faced with these situations of stepwise decline. The majority of people (88%) state that they would prefer dying at home with their family in familiar surroundings but only 20% actually achieve this goal. The majority (56%) of Americans die in the hospital and another 19% end their life in a long term care facility of some type. Some of these hospital deaths can be explained by the relatively rare sudden catastrophic event in a previously healthy individual that leads to an emergent admission to a hospital. Most deaths in America are due to the consequences of longstanding diseases. Heart disease and cancer have remained the leading causes for several decades. There are some who expire in a hospital or nursing home because they do not have the support of someone at home as the spouse is also elderly or the patient was alone with no family or close friends to provide the needed care and attention. For the most part, our mobile society has removed the younger generation from the proximity of the older generation and I have heard countless times, "I don't want to be a burden to my children...they're busy, they have their own lives to live."

Tami's mom sat with her, held her hand and they both cried together. They realized that although they had no control on the timing of the last days, they at least had come to terms with where it was not going to occur. Tami would remain in the unit where she had resided for over a decade with people who care about her, who understand her wishes and idiosyncrasies.

Her passing will be very difficult for her family, which now includes the entire staff of our unit. We all strive to maintain objectivity and professional distance from the patients for whom we care but some have left a mark, particularly this vulnerable and endearing young woman. As of the date of this writing, Tami has again achieved some stability and with luck she will make it to Christmas again this year giving both her and her mother the gift of another holiday together.

Bradley C. Buckhout, M.D.

Chapter 8
Opiates & Pain Control

Medicine makes use of many opiod products for pain control, anesthesia induction, cough suppression, control of diarrhea and treating/preventing opiod withdrawal. Many products have been used for over 150 years and unfortunately due to the euphoria/altered levels of consciousness that these agents cause they have been used recreationally for just as long. Opiate is a term classically used in pharmacology to mean a drug derived from opium. They are alkaloid compounds naturally found in the opium poppy plant, Papaver somniferum. Studies of alkaloids began in the nineteenth century when they were isolated and identified from many medicinal plants that had been used for centuries. In 1804 a German chemist isolated from opium a soporific or sleep inducing substance which he called "morphium" in honor of Morpheus, the Greek god of dreams. In German and some other Central-European languages, this is still the name of the drug. The term "morphine," used in English and French was coined by a French physicist.

The psychoactive compounds found in the opium plant include morphine, codeine, and thebaine. This latter substance has stimulating rather than depressant properties and is useful only after commercial processing. Thebaine is the raw material used in manufacturing the well known oxycodone products such as percocet and oxycontin. It is also used to produce naloxone (Narcan) which is used to block opiate effects and to reverse opiate overdosage.

Opioid, a more modern term, is used to designate all substances, both natural and synthetic, that bind to opiod receptors in the brain (including antagonists).

The term narcotic, from ancient Greek narco, meaning "to make numb" originally referred medically to any psychoactive compound with sleep-inducing properties. In the United States, it has since become associated with opiates and opiods, commonly morphine and its congener heroin (diamorphine), as well as derivatives of many of the compounds found within raw opium latex. Legally speaking, the term "narcotic" is imprecisely defined and typically has negative connotations. When used in a legal context in the U.S., a narcotic drug is one that is prohibited, such as heroin or one that is used in violation of governmental regulation.

With the recent declaration by President Trump of the national opiod crisis, emergency narcan nasal spray (opiate antidote) doses are being deployed widely to the general public to compliment the injectable version provided to emergency medical responders. All opioids, like opiates, are considered drugs of high abuse potential. They are tightly regulated but are also very profitable when sold illegally. Because of recreational use and abuse of prescriptions, the misuse of opiates lead to the deaths of between 59,000-65,000 Americans in 2016. The final tally is not complete due to needed review of death certificates to insure uniformity of definitions.

Alkaloid-containing plants have been used by humans since ancient times for therapeutic and recreational purposes. For example, medicinal plants had been known in the Mesopotamia era, around 2000 BC. The Odyssey of Homer referred to a gift given to Helen by the Egyptian queen, a drug bringing oblivion.

Bradley C. Buckhout, M.D.

It is believed that the gift was an opium-containing drug. A Chinese book on houseplants written in 1st–3rd centuries BC mentioned a medical use of Ephedra and opium poppies. Also, coca leaves have been used by South American Indians for their psychoactive effects since ancient times.

So with our experience using these substances dating back centuries, what has changed recently to lead to this public health emergency? Is it a change in society or a change in the forms of the opioids being abused? Yes, to both. It has been very challenging for physicians to practice during the last twenty-five years. At the start of this period, there were many studies showing that patients were dying in pain. Pain was not being dealt with aggressively enough and national polices were established making pain the Fifth Vital Sign (in addition to the commonly monitored blood pressure, pulse, respiratory rate and temperature). Protocols to evaluate pain levels with pain scales became mandatory. There were law suits filed for inadequate pain management. The pharmaceutical industry responded with new versions of medications that were marketed to providers as being more effective with fewer side effects and with less addictive potential than their predecessors. Many more prescriptions were written for opiates and were often prescribed in quantities that were too large and in doses that escalated beyond what was prudent. People became dependent and when their doctor stopped prescribing for them they began to doctor shop or went to the street or their family medicine cabinet for a continued supply.

Economic challenges, poor employment opportunities, the need for immediate gratification, family disintegration and many other societal changes have contributed to this dilemma. Now, the pendulum has swung to the opposite extreme. Prescribed opioids are on the decline but smuggled sources appear to be endless and there is no shortage of narcotic choices for someone seeking solace from their life situation or from withdrawal symptoms. Additionally, Fentanyl produced from chemicals similar to meperidine (demerol) was initially manufactured for its sedating properties and was used as an intravenous anesthetic for surgery. It is now well known in its patch form for chronic pain control and in lollipop and sublingual spray for severe pain relief. It is approximately 50-100 times more potent than morphine and in 2012 it was the most widely used synthetic opiod. This highly potent drug is being abused for its euphoria but it is also mixed with other opioids and its potency contributes significantly to the risk of accidental overdose.

Methadone, a synthetically produced opiod known most commonly for "methadone maintenance" clinic use to treat heroin and other opiate addiction, also has a role in pain relief. It is particularly helpful for the complex pain associated with neuropathic sources of pain but it has complicated metabolism and used inappropriately can accumulate in the body and lead to accidental overdose and toxicity.

What happens with opiate use that leads to the problems that are now plaguing so many people and leads to the death of as many as 165 people a day in our country? First, what causes people to die of opiate use? It is not usually the long term use that causes chronic health deterioration like alcohol related deaths due to eventual failure of the liver. There are some deaths from the chronic effects of opiod dependence due to the general neglect of nutrition and self care that leads to infections, accidents and other more indolent processes. But the deaths are largely due to the acute respiratory depression from a single, unintentional overdose of medication. Accumulation of the drug or a combination of the opiate with some other agent that also depresses the respiratory drive center of the brain are the cause of another group of deaths. This is the situation for which narcan has been designed and promoted. When given to someone found unresponsive with shallow or absent respirations it can be life saving by reversing the effect of the opiods that were consumed leading to the collapse. Narcan is however, a short acting medication and will often need to be repeated to prevent relapse into unconsciousness. Additional deaths, fewer in number, are related to acute lung injury from inhaled/smoked versions of the narcotics. Status epileptics (uncontrolled persistent seizures) and cardiac toxicity mostly from cocaine derivatives can also cause fatalities.

The body has four different types of opiod receptors, primarily in the brain (central nervous system) and peripheral nerves and some also in the gut and other tissues. The various opioids bind with these receptors in similar but not identical ways and will cause their effects based on the intensity of the affinity and activation of each one. The mu receptor, when stimulated is responsible for analgesia, euphoria, respiratory depression and miosis or pupillary constriction. The kappa receptor, adds to the analgesia and respiratory depression but also leads to sedation. It is important to recognize that sedation precedes suppression of respiratory drive. This fact is useful in the clinical setting when a patient has a patient controlled analgesia trigger. If accumulation of the drug is occurring, the patient becomes drowsy and will cease pressing the trigger for more drug, providing some measure of protection from an accidental overdose. Sigma receptors, when activated, are known to cause dysphoria (unpleasant sensations of dissatisfaction with life), hallucinations and in extreme cases, psychosis (loss of contact with the generally accepted reality). Delta receptors add to the euphoria and analgesia but can also lead to seizures.

When Caring Trumps Curing

When these medications are first ordered for a patient, caution is warranted as the individual's sensitivity to the effects mentioned above will need to be determined. As the body is exposed to these powerful medications it begins to adapt. The drugs are metabolized by the liver to inactivated forms for the most part, but some notably have active metabolites which may add to the analgesia or toxicity (normeperidine, a metabolite of demerol which can cause spasticity and seizures). Analgesia and sedation and a sense of euphoria or well being are the therapeutic targets being sought when these products are used medically. When they are used recreationally, euphoria is the high being chased. Respiratory depression is uncommon when these medications are used with care and titration is done judiciously.

In discussions, particularly with our World War II veterans, part of the Greatest Generation, the topic of addiction always comes up as the reason they would rather not take pain medications and would prefer to stoically endure their suffering. This attitude is a powerful, almost ubiquitous generational belief that takes some effort to dispel. Addiction is the result of long term opiod use, most commonly not for its intended purpose of pain relief but in a setting of misuse and abuse. It has been my experience, as well as the experience of most other palliative care physicians, that addiction is a rarity among palliative patients being treated appropriately for painful conditions.

Addiction is the compulsive need for and use of a habit-forming substance (such as heroin, oxycodone, nicotine, or alcohol) characterized by tolerance and by well-defined physiological symptoms upon withdrawal. This persistent compulsive use of the drug of choice continues despite the user knowing it to be harmful. The compulsion often undermines the user's ability to function normally. It can lead to loss of job, resources and relationships but persists anyway with the acquisition of the drug being the sole focus of existence. Addiction is clearly a maladaptive pattern of behavior and is not unique to opioids. It is distinctly unusual to encounter in palliative patients, and not a concern at all in a patient enrolled in hospice. As providers, we must be aware of the bias against opiod use and provide education and reassurance to patients, their families and other clinicians to be able to provide the compassionate and effective care dictated by the medical issues plaguing the patients under our care.

Tolerance is a response of the body to the continued use of the opiod class of medication. But tolerance to one opiod does not translate completely to another. In other words, with continued use of morphine for example, the body's metabolic machinery becomes more efficient and there is likely some receptor adaptation as well, so that over time the dose of medication needed to provide adequate analgesia will gradually increase. This is almost universal. This is not a sign of addiction but is a normal physiologic response. Respiratory depression diminishes, analgesia diminishes but one effect that doesn't decrease is constipation, tolerance does not develop to this opiod effect. When tolerance is not recognized or considered and medication adjusted appropriately the patient may lose control of their pain and suffer needlessly. Especially in today's environment of the "opiod crisis," the provider-patient relationship based on trust and clear goals of care is vital to insure that the medications are appropriately monitored and modified to meet the needs of the patient. In the next chapter, our patient Jeff, due to untreatable, aggressive metastatic cancer required exceptional doses of opiods and other agents to meet his stated goal: to be as pain free as possible, hopefully while being able to communicate with his family.

Chapter 9
JEFF

I have always considered myself to be a healthy guy. I played sports in high school and started on the varsity football team. College wasn't for me so I enlisted in the military when I was 20 and served two tours during the Gulf War/Desert Storm and then in a peacekeeping role in Haiti in 1995-96 with the 2nd Cav Regiment of the Army. I became a driver for one of the Humvees in my squad which had a mounted MK19 grenade launcher. We were one badass machine! During my Army days, I started smoking, not a bright thing to do but boredom and peer pressure what they are, I started and sadly I have not been able to stop.

When I got back to Arizona after the military, I was able to find work as a trucker and I have been doing that now for eleven years. I have never been married but I have had a girlfriend off and on, presently back on, maybe out of concern for what I am going through. I know my mom is worried and she gets hysterical at times so it's good that Gina is there to calm her down, something I haven't been able to do.

It was early this year, January I think, when I got sick. I had been in Minnesota hauling a load of freight from Texas and it was cold! I developed a sore throat and a fever and then this cough started that would not go away despite a bunch of over the counter cough meds. When I finally rolled back into Arizona I went to the VA and got a chest x-ray. There was something in the bottom of my left lung that they thought could be a pneumonia based on my fever and cough. I was given an antibiotic and told to come back in ten days for another chest x-ray to make sure the

Bradley C. Buckhout, M.D.

spot was going away but I was feeling better and I had to pay the bills so I took another load and headed east. During that trip, after tossing a tie down across the trailer, my right shoulder started giving me trouble. It ached deep in the shoulder blade and made lifting my arm almost impossible. I was seen in an urgent care in Ohio and was given some ibuprofen which helped with the aching, enough that I could keep driving. It was a month later when I got back to Arizona. Since the cough had not stopped completely, (of course I hadn't stopped smoking, completely) I went back to the doctor and had the requested follow up chest x-ray. The haziness in the left lung was still there. I also had an x-ray of my shoulder which didn't show anything wrong. "It must be the soft tissues" I was told, was given a different NSAID, naproxen to try and was referred to a shoulder specialist.

By the time I got in to see him in March, I couldn't lift my arm and sleeping was becoming difficult. His examination was unrevealing except that he detected my shoulder blade was sticking out a little and he suspected compression of the nerve that controls the muscle that holds it against the rib cage. I had not been able to work for several weeks and I was getting concerned about the pain. I made several trips to the emergency department and I think they thought I was just coming in for pain meds. On the fateful evening of my fourth trip the doctor felt a fleshy lump over my shoulder blade that was painful to pressure and he ordered a CT scan of the shoulder and chest.

I knew something was wrong, but to everyone's shock it was discovered that the left lung haziness had the appearance of a cancer and the lump in the shoulder blade was a large metastatic appearing tumor that was destroying the scapula. Things, after this scan, began happening quickly. I was admitted to the hospital and pulmonary, orthopedic and oncology doctors were consulted. A needle biopsy of the mass in the shoulder revealed non-small cell lung cancer. That fact meant the I had stage IV cancer, surgery was not an option and only chemotherapy and localized radiation could be offered. A PET scan was done to look for other areas where the cancer may have spread and it pointed to lesions in the bones of my low back, my left femur and the bones of my pelvis.

I was forty years old, I had just been told that I have metastatic lung cancer and that even with treatment my survival will be measured in months. I was devastated, Gina was devastated, my mom was distraught.

Focal radiation treatments to the shoulder mass were done to reduce pain. Treatments for the spine to slow progression of the tumors to reduce the risk of spinal cord compression were completed. This would hopefully decrease the risk of loss of control of the bladder, bowel or limbs. A first line chemotherapy agent was begun and although I tolerated it fairly well the cancer continued to enlarge while I was receiving the medication. I was able to be home with some nursing support during this time, but I was becoming weaker and the pain I was experiencing was becoming unbearable.

It was then that I was first introduced to the outpatient palliative care team. They were focused from the onset on helping control the bone pain that was immobilizing me. I continued seeing my oncologist but it was becoming evident that there were no effective treatments available for my very aggressive cancer. Meeting with the palliative care team was helpful, they reassured me that they were going to continue to work with me and do whatever they could to help relieve my symptoms. Traveling to the clinic was becoming an ordeal as I was having trouble putting any weight on my left leg without excruciating pain. The nurse practitioner made the suggestion that hospice be consulted so that I could stay at home and medication adjustments could be made without having to come in so often. I initially recoiled at the thought of hospice. In my mind that meant I was going to die. Someone from hospice would come out to my bedside and give me an injection of morphine and that would be the end, I would stop breathing and be gone.

With some effort the palliative team dispelled the myths and explained the kinds of services the hospice agency, under their guidance, would provide. I reluctantly agreed and returned home with Gina and my mom supported by the hospice nurses. For a few days the pain was better with frequent adjustments in the morphine pills I was receiving and I was able to get some sleep and even eat a little for the first time in a while. We were hopeful that perhaps we had reached a stable plateau on a good medication regimen where I could be comfortable, with family at home. But like before, the pain began to escalate again and my right thigh that had not been painful before now had a sharp, searing pain each time I shifted position. Initially I thought it was my imagination but it also seemed be getting larger, almost as I watched.

Returning to the VA for evaluation required the use of a stretcher van and when I arrived and the palliative team saw me they recommended admission to the hospital to evaluate the thigh swelling and to become even more aggressive with the pain control regimen. By then, I was nauseated and vomiting periodically and so an IV line was placed for some hydration, anti-vomiting medications and a hydromorphone infusion to relieve my pain. These were helpful, but not completely, so a steroid was added and an intravenous non-steroidal anti-inflammatory, ketorolac was tried. This medication combined with the others gave pain relief for a few hours. The regimen of medication I was receiving was complicated and needing frequent adjustments so the team recommended I be transferred to the CLC inpatient hospice unit where another part of the VA hospice team would assume my care.

I had discussed Jeff's case with the outpatient palliative team and was aware that he was being transferred to our unit with very aggressive metastatic lung cancer. He was young, only 40 years old and had been diagnosed just six months ago. His symptoms first appeared just months before that. We are very familiar with caring for end of life patients due to a variety of conditions, but they are usually at least twenty years older than Jeff and are often twice his age. In general, those veterans are more frail with many issues contributing to their declining health. Jeff was young and healthy save for this malignancy. He was not a diabetic, did not have hypertension nor vascular disease, his kidneys were healthy and he had not smoked long enough or heavily enough to have significant impairment of his lung function. He could live a long time, relatively speaking, perhaps exceeding the usual 6-9 month prognosis for his widely metastatic cancer.

When I arrived in the CLC, I was pleased to find that I would have a room to myself. There was a view out the window to a patch of grass and then the parking lot, always active, something to watch instead of the blank ceiling or the pathetic stuff on TV. I was having trouble concentrating on television anyway due to the constant pain in my hip and back and shoulder.

The doctor, with two PA students, the nurse practitioner and the pharmacist who I knew from the outpatient clinic arrived soon after I was situated in bed. I was on a special air mattress to keep me from getting pressure sores. I could not easily change position due to pain and I had already lost much of my muscle and fat padding over my bony prominences due to the disease and loss of

Bradley C. Buckhout, M.D.

appetite. Despite the seriousness of my condition, they all were confident that things would get better and they would find a combination of medications that would let me rest peacefully. They made me feel hopeful and before they were done with their exam they had me laughing for the first time in a long while. They spent time talking with Gina and mom too and offered them reassurance that they would be available to help us through this process.

I was leaving the hospital with my hydromorphone drip running at 3 mg/hr but I still had required bolus doses of 1 mg at least once an hour all last night. The team in the CLC hospice was aware of this and almost immediately upon arrival in the CLC increased the rate of my infusion and I was given a PCA button to use to give me more control over my medication dosing. The PCA is a patient controlled analgesia trigger that causes the IV pump to administer a fixed dose of pain medication each time the button is pushed, as long as the request is outside a preset lockout interval since the last dose was given. The nice thing about this button is when I had pain, I didn't have to wait for a nurse to respond to my call light, the pump medicated me automatically.

Jeff's cancer was very aggressive. He had been seen by our oncology team and had been given local radiation therapy to his shoulder and spine, four courses of carboplatin + paclitaxil. This is a palliative treatment designed to slow progression of the cancer to reduce symptoms but would not be curative. The cancer unfortunately, had not responded to these agents and had actually grown during therapy. As is often the case, chemotherapy added new symptoms to the pain he was already experiencing. His hair began to depart...in chunks. He developed dry mouth with sores on his tongue and lips making drinking and eating difficult. He had a cough for days after each infusion and the coughing racked him with pain in his shoulder and his thoracic spine where there was another bone being destroyed. Thankfully, the tumor was growing towards the skin and not inward. Had it grown inward, it could have led to pressure on the spinal cord and possibly paralysis. Also worse after treatment was the feeling of exceptional fatigue and achiness, like he had the flu x3. That is why he had finally come to the hospital and then to an inpatient hospice unit. He was suffering at home and more intensive symptom management was necessary. His pain was constant and severe. Short acting pain medications were not able to stay ahead of his pain so long acting oral morphine had been started at home. When he was admitted to the hospital, intravenous hydromorphone was started to give more constant drug levels with the goal of more constant pain relief. This derivative is significantly more potent than its parent compound, morphine, requiring smaller volumes of medication for equivalent pain relief. He previously had a port surgically implanted under the skin of his chest for access to his blood vessels for chemotherapy. Now this port would be utilized to provide medications for symptom control.

Hydromorphone (Dilaudid) has the same side effect concerns as other opiates: sedation, followed by respiratory depression and constipation to which tolerance does not develop. In our experience it causes less of the confusion, muscle jerking and hallucinations that we see occasionally with morphine. Morphine is considered the parent compound, the central pillar of opiate therapy. All of the conversions of this group of medications are based on their morphine equivalent daily dose (MEDD). There are numerous calculators available to assist with conversions and on our unit, we always double check our math with another team member, most commonly a clinical pharmacist. Sometimes the reason for conversion is a change in the patient's condition. If, for example renal function begins to deteriorate, accumulation of morphine metabolites can become problematic so conversion to an agent that is less dependent on kidney excretion would be wise.

The nurses were in my room a lot. They could see in my face that I wasn't comfortable and to their credit they did the best they could to reposition me and to offer the medications that were available. They had obviously dealt with sick patients before. My mom and Gina were constant companions during this transition to the new unit. I know they were concerned about me but I think they were worried about the care I would get in the CLC. The unknown is always frightening and I was going to be cared for by another new team of doctors and nurses, people that I didn't know. My experience with the outpatient palliative team and the docs in the hospital had been good. Who was this new team, would they be as aggressive with my pain medications, would they listen? I could understand their concern. Heck, I was a little nervous at first, but everyone here has put me at ease and they are clearly trying to help.

The doctor was in again with the pharmacist and the nurse practitioner. They are openly discussing pain control options with all of us. Mom and Gina would like me to be as alert as possible so that my days are not totally lost with me in a drug induced haze. It is clear to me that the time I have left is rapidly dwindling. I am pretty certain that I won't be here for Christmas this year and I don't want to spend all my time asleep either. But the pain in my shoulder, hip and low back are something that I can't describe. There is this dull pressure, throbbing when I am laying perfectly still. I can tell how fast my heart is beating by the pulsing of this pain. When I move, even a little, that pain is overwhelmed by this intense hot electric jolt in my shoulder or hip that takes my breath away. I am ashamed to cry, but there have been times when I couldn't control the tears. I really hate to do that because it really upsets my family.

When Caring Trumps Curing

It has been said that serious illnesses sometimes have positive effects, I never understood that until now. My illness and the love and concern from Mom and Gina for me, has brought them together and has healed the old wounds that they were both carrying. I really wish we could have come up with a better way, but for the time being I am happy with this result. They are here for me but I know this is really draining both of them. Because they are helping each other now, they can take turns in their vigil so one can rest while the other stays with me.

I have been in bed now for about ten days, I can't remember exactly, the days are beginning to run together. There is no calendar in the room…thank goodness. It really doesn't matter anyway. I am here, there is nothing I can do about it. The cancer is in charge. It has my fate in its claws and it is literally gnawing on my bones. My mom has had a really hard time with this. She is a lot better than she was in the clinic when she used to sob uncontrollably whenever I had to go back for another appointment. I don't think she is accepting this any better than she was. Maybe she has just gotten numb to the emotional drain that a parent must feel when their child is dying.

I don't consider myself a child, I'm 40 years old. I've been to war, which I survived, despite being shot at and nearly blown up by a roadside IED. Now, I'm dying from the cigarettes. What a stupid thing to die from. It was cool when I started and like every other smoker, I was certain all of those warnings were for other people. I was indestructible. But apparently twenty years of inhaling the addicting toxins was too much for my lungs to recover from. To a mother though, her child is always her child and there is no resolving the disconnect that their child will not be around as long as she will. She was all alone until Gina came back. Dad has been gone for three years and it was hard on her losing him so suddenly. I had already been gone for almost 20

Bradley C. Buckhout, M.D.

years from their house and when I moved in with Gina, initially to just share expenses six years ago, they were not happy. Gina, of course was not good enough for their first child and only son. How many times has that been said in homes across this country?

In addition to the dilaudid drip we applied a lidocaine transdermal patch to the skin of the thigh, where that pain was localized. He was also able to get doses of lorazepam, an anti-anxiety agent as needed for the stress he was feeling. He understood clearly the gravity of his situation and had come to the realization that his life would most likely end here...in this room.

His PRN (given as needed per patient request) use of medications and responses to them were monitored multiple times each day. He was also still on dexamethasone, a steroid that is useful as an adjunct for bone pain. Haloperidol, an effective treatment for nausea and also for delirium was available as needed and he was also receiving ketorolac, a potent pain relieving non-steroidal anti-inflammatory. This medication is usually utilized for short term, most often in emergency rooms and after surgery. It is a good analgesic but it has a significant risk of ulcerating the lining of the gastrointestinal tract, causing abdominal pain and bleeding. It had been discovered in Jeff's case the pain relief that it provided was of quick onset and remarkably effective for several hours after each IV dose. We discussed the risks among the team and with Jeff and his family. They were all in favor of continuing the ketorolac (toradol) even though we were already well beyond the recommended duration of therapy, because they could see him relax after each IV push of the medication.

Nights were particularly bad. He had difficulty falling to sleep and then if he moved the electric bolts of pain would have him fully awake. His medication doses, both the constant infusion and the prn bolus doses were adjusted frequently. We were able to achieve sufficient pain control that the welcome oblivion of sleep was, on some nights obtained. When I saw him on day six he was rested. He was eating breakfast and was able to move his legs, without staff assistance. This was a dramatic improvement and he expressed his gratitude with the comfort, however temporary it might be.

I finally got uninterrupted sleep last night, five hours of peaceful escape from reality. Unfortunately, when I awoke this morning it is apparent that I have not been stuck in a nightmare. I am still here in this hospital room, hooked up to a potent narcotic, stuck in bed because my legs cannot be trusted and if I challenge them I know they will strike me down with agonizing pain. Gina is with me. So this is not a complete nightmare. Why does she stay? What can I give her now? She says she loves me…

Gina comes back to sit on the side of my bed with a grin, "What was that movie with Ryan O'Neal and Ali McGraw, from the '70's?"

"What, you're going to challenge me with trivia while my brain is full of dilaudid? Not very fair, babe."

"Oh right, sorry Jeff, but you always have amazed me with your obscure trivial facts."

"That's OK dear, remember, love means never having to say you're sorry. That by the way is a huge clue."

"Ah yes, Love Story. I don't remember much about the movie but I do remember it was about a young girl who died of cancer and her boyfriend. Lot's of crying at the end."

Bradley C. Buckhout, M.D.

She stopped, her eyes welling with tears. "I hope somehow, our story ends differently."

Day 7, labs appeared in Jeff's record this morning. We generally don't check lab work in our hospice patients. We really don't need to know how badly the body's various organ systems are failing as we are not likely to intervene to correct the problems that are developing. By this point in the dying process, our purpose is to address only the symptoms that are distressing patients. The lab work rarely offers information that we can use to help. We then noticed that the labs had been ordered by Jeff's oncologist, apparently in preparation for another chemotherapy infusion. We called the oncologist and discussed with him that Jeff was now in hospice and that his functional status was so poor that chemotherapy would not be indicated and would likely make him worse.

Chemotherapy, even when done for palliation, is usually reserved for patients who are at least able to spend some time out of bed. The effects of chemotherapy often are severely debilitating and a patient must have some measure of strength and reserve to be able to withstand the treatment. We then spent time discussing with Jeff, Gina and his mother, the conversation we had with the oncologist and he readily agreed that he wouldn't be able to tolerate the side effects of another round of chemo. We did discuss the possibility of doing focal radiation treatments to his hip, but also that logistically, since he was on such high doses of opioids that transferring him to the outside treatment center would be a very challenging ordeal. Jeff's response was that the current treatments he was receiving were giving better pain control than he had gotten when they radiated him before. We had, in this conversation, taken further palliative therapies off the table.

When Caring Trumps Curing

We have a unique philosophy concerning hospice treatment not shared by most community facilities. We allow concurrent care with the medical oncologists, radiation oncologists, surgeons and other specialties after a veteran has committed to hospice care. So, while in hospice, we have had patients receive palliative chemo and radiation treatments with the goal of symptom management. If the patient desires, we will treat urinary infections, if pneumonia is causing respiratory distress we will start antibiotics and respiratory treatments if needed. It is clear that this philosophy has reduced pain and fear and has allowed patients to live much longer and perhaps achieve some uncompleted goals before they die. It also makes the suggestion to consider hospice care less of a black and white, either/or proposition. Patients can chose "one from column A and one from column B" and it is my impression that acceptance of the hospice care team occurs earlier in the disease process, before the symptom burden becomes overwhelming. There is a huge quality of life benefit for the patients selecting this route.

Our meeting with Jeff, Gina and his mom on day nine revealed a pattern of fairly comfortable nights but early morning awakening with severe pain. During the day he had been awake and conversant and able to eat some pizza that Gina brought in. We altered the ketorolac dosing to every 6 hours and changed the timing of the doses so that he would receive some at 4 a.m. before he had been waking with pain the last few days. We again discussed the risk of GI bleeding but because it was still effective in providing rapid pain relief they were all willing to accept the risks. There was also a change in emphasis by his mom, "Please do what you need to do to make him comfortable, even if it means he is going to sleep more." Prior to this request, they had wanted him to be awake and alert enough for them to spend quality time with him. This is a very common dilemma that we face and discussions with patients and families regularly address this fine balancing act. The patient's needs are considered first and obviously are the most important, but when treating a hospice patient we are treating the entire group that surrounds him, the people who he considers his support. Family, friends, church members, biker buddies, AA sponsors, any number of combinations who are all on this journey too, need to be considered.

In Jeff's case, we were being very aggressive with his dilaudid and yet he was able to remain awake and be conversant without much evidence of mental clouding or confusion. By day eleven, when we stopped to check on him, Gina reported that, "Everything is pretty good". Jeff woke briefly, while we were in the room, waved and was observed to be repositioning himself in bed. Earlier that morning, he had been able to tolerate a bed bath.

Day 13, ketorolac frequency is increased to every 4 hours and Jeff had a quiet night. He was able to have a bowel movement with the use of a small enema. This is a vitally important bodily function that is significantly impaired by opiates of all types. He had been receiving bowel stimulants and stool softeners since before his hospitalization and continued monitoring to insure he did not get constipated adding to his discomfort is another important part of palliative and hospice protocols.

Day 15, Jeff wants to get up in the wheelchair to be able to go outside!

Day 19, his hydromorphone doses had been incrementally increased in response to the recorded prn doses that he was requiring during each twenty-four hour period. He is awake this morning and appears relaxed and comfortable compared to three days ago. He was able to sit on the side of the bed and visit with friends. Because of the high volumes of fluids being delivered intravenously carrying the pain medications he was having to urinate frequently and was having trouble positioning the urinal. At his request, a catheter was placed in his bladder to prevent incontinence. When we visit today, he is awake and drinking juice with his head resting on his stuffed raccoon, his legs elevated on a mound of pillows. On the wall is a sign, written in a woman's hand "Push the GREEN Button". Taped to the TV, another in similar writing, "Push the Pain Button". His mom tells us that Gina had to leave to go back home. Her mother has just been hospitalized and was discovered to have cancer. Gina wanted to make sure Jeff didn't forget to use is PCA button while she was gone.

Day 22, Jeff is asleep this morning and his mom, at the bedside reported that he had a good night but awoke with his usual 5 a.m. hip/leg pain. His respirations were even and unlabored at fifteen breaths a minute while sleeping. His hydromorphone dose by now, was dramatically higher than is required for our usual hospice patients. In most people, sedation and respiratory depression would be of significant concern at his dose. The key to recall in Jeff's case is that he was a young healthy male who had developed a significant tolerance over time to the effects of opiods, both for pain control and also undesirable side effects. His ketorolac is now being given every 3 hours and he is again using lidocaine patches on the most painful locations. He is also able to use lorazepam 1 mg IV every 3 hours if necessary. We also gave a dose of zolidronic acid, a bisphosphonate medication, routinely used for osteoporosis treatment that can give prompt relief from bone pain from metastatic bone damage. His goal remains pain control. The ability to be awake and communicate is now of secondary importance. We are still achieving this for the most part, some days his pain is 3 out of 10 on the pain scale but still with flares to 10 out of 10 randomly.

Bradley C. Buckhout, M.D.

Day 28, Gina is still with her mom but Jeff was able to talk with her by phone last evening. His mother reports that he woke this morning trembling from the pain. She really wants his suffering to end and is OK with him being asleep most of the time if that's what it takes to give him more relief. He would like to go outside and nursing is making arrangements for this to happen, in his bed if they can't get him safely into a chair. A family member is bringing in a photo collage for the wall at the foot of his bed. Jeff's mom went home to get cleaned up and while she was away the nursing staff assembled a large enough team to accomplish his trip outdoors. There is a patio, not contaminated by smokers, with a garden and trees outside of his room, not a long trip by bed. It was August in Phoenix, the temperature was well over 100 degrees, so this was not going to be a long excursion. Unfortunately, Jeff's mom returned when his bed was out of the room and she immediately assumed the worst...he had died while she was gone. She passed me in the hallway, frantic and in tears, "Where is he, where is my son?" We located him as the staff was wheeling him down the hallway back to his room, she was relieved but upset that she had not been able to accompany him on what would be his last trip outside.

Day 30, we had added low dose oral methadone to his hydromorphone regimen with the theory that it affects other opiod receptors and can improve receptor sensitivity that diminishes after long term opiod use. Unfortunately, Jeff was beginning to have difficulty swallowing some of his medications and so we began to alter routes of delivery where that was possible. He was resting more comfortably and appeared to be dozing for longer periods but he was still easily arousable and was able to answer questions coherently.

Jeff's case was truly an outlier for all of us caring for him and we had frequent conversations with the remainder of the palliative care providers for their suggestions. There were discussions about the "ceiling opiod dose," a dose beyond which only side effects are increased, not pain relief. The concept makes sense physiologically. At some serum level of drug all of the available receptors will be bound and no further effect on symptoms would be expected. While agreeing with the concept, patient's respond in unique ways. With each dose increase, Jeff had an incremental decrease in pain, at least for some hours before further titration was needed. There was also consideration given to adding ketamine, an agent used most commonly as an anesthetic for surgery, but when given in low doses it can serve as an adjunct in pain control. This could have perhaps added to his comfort but we have had no experience with this medication and the studies in the medical literature on its use are limited and the side effects were worrisome. Out of body experiences, dysphoria and hallucinations being reported frequently enough that the potential for tormenting Jeff with these in his last days made the benefit/risk tilted too far toward the latter, particularly since he had reported bad dreams and seeing bugs on the wall the previous night.

Day 34, Jeff is sleeping, breathing easily and appears to be at peace. Gina has gotten back from the time spent with her mother and she is at the bedside. "He had a good night as far as pain but while he was half asleep he was having conversations with people who weren't here," she said. "He wasn't freaked out by it and when I touched him and asked who he was talking to he would say, nobody". She looked at me, "What's that all about?"

"With the amount of medications he is on that can affect his brain function and perception we are all frankly very surprised that he is awake at all and able to still communicate meaningfully with you and his mother. He is truly a case for the record books! Hallucinations are certainly not surprising based just on the medications but we also see this frequently as people approach the end of their life. Conversations with loved ones who have gone before are common, almost as if they have come to welcome the person to the next existence."

"I have heard of that and seen it in the movies but do you think it really happens?" Gina asked.

"We obviously don't know what is going on in someone's mind but I have been in rooms while patients carry on conversation with their grandmother or father or someone they miss, clearly rekindling a relationship. It has been my experience that these exchanges don't provoke anxiety and actually patients often seem calmer once these interactions have occurred. When it happens it is usually in the last days of life. Some providers consider it a terminal delirium as brain functions start their final decline. Indeed some people become inconsolably restless in the last days and hours and require medications to calm them so they don't fall out of bed and injure themselves".

"It doesn't seem to bother him and like I said he just seemed to be talking with someone I couldn't see. I don't think we need to try and stop it especially if it is preparing him for an easier transition to whatever is next," Gina reasonably concluded.

Today, for the first time, there was some evidence of wheezing and his breathing was more labored than it had been during the month he had been with us. Breathing treatments with albuterol were ordered when needed. As the day progressed, he became more restless, wringing his hands, trying to reposition, wincing with every movement. His hydromorphone was increased further as was his lorazepam infusion to try to provide him with comfort so that he could rest. His mother noted that he had slept probably a total of four hours the previous evening and was fidgety throughout the night. The clinical appearance was that he was in a terminal delirium which occurs in as many as 85% of patients as they enter the last phase of the dying process. Haloperidol is often very helpful in reducing the hallucinations and bringing a calming affect to the mind that is no longer processing input very well.

Day 38, there has been a change today in Jeff's condition. His skin is warm and flushed and his breathing has a wet congested sound to it and he is having difficulty swallowing and clearing his secretions. His wet tracheal-pharyngal respirations have been dubbed the 'death rattle' as they are a sign that the swallowing mechanism, a very basic reflex is failing. Usually, within hours after that reflex ceases the automatic drive to breathe ends and shortly after life itself ends. The heart beat will persist, but not for long in the absence of oxygen. Jeff's mother, sister, brother-in-law and Gina were all at the bedside, evidence of the emotional exhaustion they were all feeling was apparent. Jeff, on his back with his head elevated, lay not stirring, in bed. He was breathing rapidly and audibly but did not appear to be in distress. We spoke with the family softly, to not disturb him.

"How much longer can this go on? It's becoming really hard to watch my son like this. We've been here five weeks now, when will this finally be over?"

"Your son has been incredibly strong. None of us can fathom the tolerance that he has shown to the amount of medication we have given him to try to allow him some comfort and quality time with you all."

"We very much appreciate all of your efforts and caring. We know your team has done everything you could and we are thankful that we had this time with him," Gina added, her arm around Jeff's mom's shoulders.

Bradley C. Buckhout, M.D.

"The changes we are seeing suggest that he probably has an infection that is overwhelming what is left of his defenses. His breathing pattern makes us think that he is likely not going to last the rest of today. I'd like to say I'm sorry, but with all that you and Jeff have been through I think his last breath will finally bring some relief to all of you. Psychologically, I know you have all been preparing for the end, even though it is a totally unacceptable proposition to consider. People talk about losing hope and what that does to a patient and their family as they go through any chronic illness. Jeff never lost hope through this ordeal and neither have you, but the meaning of hope has changed with the changing information and the progress of his disease."

At the beginning when the lump was first discovered; I hope this isn't cancer. Then when the doctor raised that ugly specter; I hope the doctor is wrong. When the biopsy proved that it was cancer; I hope it hasn't spread to other places and when there was evidence that it had; I hope the chemotherapy can cure this. When chemo was started; I hope it won't make me sick and make me lose my hair. When it became apparent that the cancer was not responding to treatment; I hope I won't suffer, I hope someone will care, I hope I won't be alone, I hope they will tell me the truth. Now as we near the end; I hope he won't suffer, I hope he won't linger, I hope it will occur quickly and painlessly.

Our team left the room to care for other patients and we were soon summoned back to Jeff's room by his bedside nurse, "It's over." We returned and he was silent. Gina was on one side of the bed holding his hand tears dropping on his face. His mother sobbing softly on the other side of the bed with a bottle of Biotene spray in her hand. She looked up and said, "He was breathing through his mouth and it was so dry, so I sprayed some of this and then he stopped breathing...it was so sudden."

When Caring Trumps Curing

"It wasn't because of the spray that he stopped," I reassured her.

"I know."

"But if that was all it took to finally give him peace, we should have tried that weeks ago." I replied trying to lighten the mood.

Thankfully, it was accepted as intended and we shared a final chuckle with this family at the end of a very draining journey. They were in a sense fortunate, they had quality time with Jeff before he passed away. Time to share hopes and wishes and memories, but the death of a child is never something a parent should have to experience.

Bradley C. Buckhout, M.D.

Chapter 10
Don

Doc:

I want the truth, lately I can be lying in bed and my tumors will start bleeding for no apparent reason. I'm no doctor but it tells me my days on this earth are becoming shorter. Am I correct? Please be honest and tell me the truth. If I am correct, all I hope for is that I go in my sleep. If I don't that's OK too, I'm just hoping. Whenever I am awake all my nose does is run and run and run. It's driving me crazy. Like I already said, it tells me that my days are growing shorter. Nurses are having trouble getting gauze to stay in place and I'm glad because when they do, it's too tight and very uncomfortable. My friends keep telling me to get better I know they mean well but they should know that's impossible with what's wrong with me.

This was a note to me written by Don, a 64 year old Army veteran of the Vietnam War whose life after the war had not gone well. He had written the note because he is no longer able to speak, having undergone surgery to remove a tumor near his vocal cords. The tumor turned out to be a squamous cell carcinoma. Aggressive resection, taking his entire larynx with some of the surrounding tissue including 1/2 of his thyroid gland was done in an attempt to cure the cancer. A myocutaneous flap from

When Caring Trumps Curing

his upper chest was rotated to cover the resulting hole in his neck in February 2016.

This kind of cancer is most frequently found in people who smoke and drink, activities which Don did habitually. Divorce ended his marriage and he was estranged from his son and the rest of the family. Chronic back pain made employment difficult and Don had not held a job with any regularity. Depression and suicidal thoughts as a result of these life stresses led to a hospitalization in 2008. Throat pain and swallowing difficulty in May 2015 were evaluated and he was discovered to have a gastric ulcer and Barrett's esophagus, a common finding in people with reflux and a possible precursor to esophageal cancer. Treatment for these problems did not relieve his swallowing problems so a CT scan of the neck was completed in November 2015 and a mass was discovered which lead to biopsy and the surgery at the Mayo Hospital. A PET scan done at the time showed evidence of tumor in the lymph nodes in both sides of his neck which indicated that the cancer had already spread. Even though the surgery he had undergone was very aggressive, disfiguring and life changing it would not be curative. I am not sure that Don was completely aware of what lay ahead for him when he agreed to have the surgery. It behooves patients to speak with the medical providers to whom they are entrusting their care and ultimately their life. Some physicians do not do a very good job informing and educating people about the options they have and what the realistic outcomes may be as a result of the treatment selected. As a family doctor I spent a great deal of my time with patients explaining to them what specialists had not made clear.

After his surgery Don elected to not undergo radiation to the regional nodes but did elect palliative chemotherapy. A feeding tube had been placed through his abdominal wall as he was unable to eat or speak following the surgery. Follow up PET scans in June showed new metastases in the lungs despite the chemotherapy. He had begun eating again and requested removal of his feeding tube in July. Then in November a recurrent tumor was found along the right side of the neck incision. It was recommended that he return to Mayo for consideration of further surgery but he declined.

In February 2017 he was no longer able to swallow and he was admitted to the hospital to have a PEG tube placed again. This time he was seen by the palliative care service who arranged for hospice support at home and he was discharged with their assistance. He unfortunately did not do well. His support was limited as he was relying only on a friend and the hospice team. Delivery of supplies had not been timely so he had gone days without tube feedings. The hospice service had taken him off the fentanyl patch which was controlling his neck pain. It is a much more expensive medication which few hospice services will provide. They had ordered a long acting morphine as a replacement. Unfortunately, these cannot be crushed and put down a feeding tube because their timed delivery mechanism is disrupted and too much drug is absorbed rapidly. Since the tube was his only route of intake, he had not taken any sustained release morphine and therefore had not slept for two days when he was admitted to our unit.

If teens had the opportunity to sit with Don for a few minutes I'm fairly certain they would reassess the cool image that smoking cigarettes seems to convey to them. Don is thin, to the point of being skeletal. His record indicates 103 pounds, a loss of 64 pounds since his diagnosis. I'm certain this is due to the wasting that is common to cancer sufferers as the tumors aggressively consume nutrients being provided to keep the body alive. In addition, his intake has suffered since he can no longer swallow. For a time, he requested that his feeding tube be removed while he attempted to maintain some semblance of normalcy by eating by mouth even with the risk of choking and aspirating the food and drink into his lungs. Because his pharynx had been surgically invaded and the normal patterns of mucus drainage altered, he has a constant purulent appearing drainage coming from both nostrils. It has become so persistent that he is no longer aware of it. This is a bit disconcerting as one sits and talks with him and the strands of snot dangling from his nostrils grow steadily longer until the weight is too great and they plunge to land on whatever is below; his writing pad or chest or lap. When I first met him I spied a box of tissue which I offered to him. He was initially puzzled but then got the hint and wiped away the nasal mucus strand before it made its plunge. What we tend to forget is that during the day, when we are healthy our nasal passages, mouth and throat produce over a quart of mucus that we routinely swallow. As you have certainly experienced if you have something that irritates those membranes, a cold, allergies, sinus infection, spicy foods, the production can increase dramatically. That was clearly the situation with Don.

Sadly, this is not the most disturbing feature of Don's appearance. He has a tracheostomy, a hole with a cannula in his lower throat through which he breathes. This opening also produces mucus in large quantities and when he coughs he expels large volumes of this tenacious often blood tinged stringy fluid. If he has sufficient warning he can catch it with a wash cloth but on occasion the cough is so sudden that he cannot react in time. As providers, remaining nimble when working with Don is important for infection control reasons as well as avoiding the "ick factor" of being splattered with his secretions.

Flanking this opening on both sides of his neck are large fungating, ulcerated masses with areas of black tissue and rivulets of blood in some of the fissures on the surface. There is the faint but

Bradley C. Buckhout, M.D.

very distinctive odor of necrosis surrounding Don when one approaches within a few feet. These are tumor masses that have eroded through the skin of the surgical incisions and similar to a car accident draw the eye almost irresistibly to them.

Don has a hand mirror with which he inspects these masses frequently, monitoring them for signs of bleeding. Last night the left one bled for almost twenty minutes before it could be stopped. He keeps a stack of gauze nearby so that he can apply pressure to try to manage these disfiguring masses on his own. Again, the theme of maintaining control over the ever diminishing part of life that is still not out of control is evident. All of this was a remarkable visage to encounter when we met Don for the first time. His appearance, shocking to someone not used to dealing with head and neck cancer patients, was even for those who are in the field, dramatically disquieting. But what Don did as we began our interview gave me some hope that working with him would not be something to dread. After introducing myself and explaining my role in the CLC the conversation eventually got to the question, "So with all that's been going on, how are you feeling?"

He began to write in his small but legible script on his note pad. 'I feel like S_ _ _'.

So we begin a game of Hangman. "Is there an H?" I ask. He shakes his head, nasal mucus swinging precariously. He then completes the word, "S O U P".

"You feel like soup?" I attempt to clarify, somewhat amazed to see that despite his predicament his sense of humor is apparently still intact. Don smiled and tapped the word with his pen. Humor, even in the face of life threatening illness, when it is clear that the end will soon be here, remains an important factor for improving

When Caring Trumps Curing

the quality of the remaining time for the patient and his loved ones. In appropriate situations, it can humanize the interactions between the providers and the patient and break the tension of the initial encounters and create a more personal alliance between the doctor and patient. I frequently meet a patient for the first time with one of our nurses who is also a veteran. He has the advantage of this automatic military camaraderie but he then augments that with his introduction.

"My name is Silas, I'll be your nurse for the day. If you keep your expectations low, I won't disappoint you." After the laughter subsides the patient will then turn towards me inquisitively. I have to preface the next exchange by letting you know that I dress in casual business attire; no white doctor coat, no necktie but often a stethoscope draped around my neck.

"So, are you the doctor here?" they ask.

"Yes, sir. They took my mop away again, so I'm your doctor."

Hospice care seeks both to minimize the discomfort of dying and enhance the quality of life during the final weeks or months. Humor is one means for accomplishing that. On the other hand, too much humor, or misplaced humor, can trivialize the situation, deny the reality, and prevent more direct communication. There are some patients and some interactions where the use of humor is not well received, particularly if the interactions with previous providers have been contentious or difficult. In those instances, building rapport, beginning to understand the importance of the issues being faced and understanding the patient's personality and sources of strength and support are vital.

Part of the training in palliative and hospice care has to do with having difficult conversations with patients and families. Conversations when the reality of prognosis, treatment options, goals of care and indeed for the remaining life, fears and anxieties are brought up for discussion. These discussions may occur over several visits as conditions and situations change and during these frank talks revelations about the inner core of the patient are revealed. A technique commonly used for these conversations is known by its acronym: SPIKES.

Set Up: The provider, prior to beginning this conversation must thoroughly review the record and be familiar with the care received to the present and what information has been imparted to the patient by the previous providers. The conversation should occur where some semblance of privacy can be assured. There should be little chance for distractions and interruptions. The TV is off, cell phone and pager muted, a place for everyone to sit at the same level and all of the interested parties present, strictly based on the preference of the patient. It is of note that certain cultures do not want the patient, particularly an elder, involved in conversations about death as it may call the spirits to hasten the passing. Other cultures want the entire family involved. The provider needs to determine the preferences before beginning so as to not insult or alienate the people for whom care is being offered. Introductions of all of the people involved should be made and roles explained. It can be difficult to establish trust quickly but the provider will be more successful if some rapport can be established by demonstrating an understanding of the situation, empathy and a willingness to listen and to take the time necessary to engage with the patient and family members.

Perception: "before you tell, ask". That is, before discussing the medical findings, the clinician should use open-ended questions to create a reasonably accurate picture of how the patient perceives the medical situation, what it is and how serious it is. For example, "What have you been told about your medical situation so far?" or "What is your understanding of the reasons that you have been transferred to this unit?" Based on the responses the provider can correct misinformation and tailor the bad news to what the patient understands. It can also accomplish the important task of determining if the patient or family is engaging in any variation of illness denial: wishful thinking, omission of essential but unfavorable medical details of the illness, or unrealistic expectations of treatment.

Invitation: Before the discussion proceeds, it must be determined how much the patient or family want to know. Some, as above, don't want information shared directly with the patient. Some patients are unable to accept the amount of information, particularly bad news at one time. It is not unusual to have this process take several meetings and it is often necessary to reassess the patient's perception of his situation at the start of each session.

Knowledge: It is important to determine what the patient understands about the disease process and what they have heard about treatments and prognosis. I note what they "have heard" as a very important distinction from what the chart says they "have been told". It is quite amazing when I ask why someone has come to our unit, for hospice care, how often they profess no knowledge that they have cancer. If they are aware, often their understanding is that the palliative treatment they are receiving will be curative and that the plan is for them to get some therapy, become stronger and go home. Once there is an understanding about the information the patient possesses then corrections, additions and discussions can ensue, based on the amount of information desired.

Empathy: After disclosing information that is negative, allowing time for the patient to process is important. Doctors tend to want to talk, to educate, to reassure but sometimes silence is therapeutic. Acknowledging and identifying the patient's emotional response validates that what they are feeling is a natural reaction to a stressful, frightening, incomprehensible situation in which they are now engulfed.

Summary/Strategy: In a tactful way, reviewing what has been learned, what the future holds, what is to be done from the patient's perspective insures that the patient comprehends their challenges and strategies for moving forward. What the provider must convey during this phase of the conversation is that the patient will not be abandoned. The phrase "there is nothing more that can be done" does not apply to the palliative care mode of practice. The palliative care/hospice team has many facets and they are all enrolled to provide the best quality of life no matter what the duration.

During these discussions, an interpersonal connection begins to be forged and with that, some trust and comfort in communication. It is then that the power of humor, smiles, laughter can become part of the therapeutic armamentarium in the coming battles that the patient will face. "Laughter is the best medicine," said Mary Kay Morrison, president of the Association for Applied and Therapeutic Humor, "unless you have diarrhea". She has studied the impact humor has on the brain and on the stress levels of patients in their final days. The right humor at the right time, she says, can infuse the brain with pleasurable hits of the stimulant dopamine, decrease muscle tension and anxiety in the body's nervous system, and momentarily diminish feelings of pain, anger or sadness.

Don had refused further palliative chemo or radiation therapy and had completed advanced directives; he was praised for his foresight. He did not want any life sustaining treatments and had come to the CLC-hospice to live out his remaining days, preferably not in pain. He walks short distances about his room and is seen rearranging the stuff scattered over his bed that he brought from home. During encounters he was often rummaging through bags piled on the floor looking for…what? He wanted desperately some uninterrupted sleep, a commodity often rare in a hospital, but perhaps achievable in our hospice unit. He requested continuation of his tube feedings and he also wanted a supply of "comfort liquids", apple, orange and tomato juices for their taste. He knew that he would not be able to swallow much of them but the flavor and sensation were comforting.

His pain in his throat, neck and back was constant so it was very clear that a long acting opiate was needed. Many of the traditional sustained action tablets cannot be broken or the time release feature is disrupted and too much medication is released at once. This is one of the reasons that oxycontin has become such an abused drug on the streets and is also one of the reasons it has some of the highest overdose fatalities associated with its abuse. Nearly 500,000 Americans have died of drug overdoses from 2000 to 2014. Misusing, diverting prescriptions or combining medications obtained illegally have been the greatest contributors. Between 2013 & 2014 there has been a 9% increase in deaths from natural and semi-synthetic opioids, the class to which oxycontin belongs. Heroin deaths increased 26% and Fentanyl, the most prescribed of the synthetic opioids was associated with a 90% increase during that same period.(2)

Fentanyl relies on subcutaneous fat stores for even absorption and distribution of the medication as it is released from its transdermal patch. In hospice patients fat stores have usually dwindled. Body temperatures vary which may alter absorption and vasoconstriction of the skin blood vessels may make absorption unreliable so we don't use this product in the last weeks of life when reliable symptom management is of great importance.

Bradley C. Buckhout, M.D.

Our choice was methadone. It will provide quick pain relief and will also provide long term sustained drug levels to aid in pain control. Methadone tablets may be crushed without disturbing their mechanism and it is also available as liquid that can be given through his PEG tube or orally as long as he is able to take small amounts of fluid. To aid in pain control during titration of the methadone, Don was provided rapid acting morphine to be used for breakthrough pain.

With initiation of the new medication regimen, Don became delirious and his medications were adjusted further. Interactions during his second week in the CLC revolved around whether he would ever be able to go back home…he thought, for a time, that he might want to try it again (independence, a difficult thing to relinquish). After we discussed that he could not be alone safely and that the hospice team could not be present all the time he decided to remain under our care.

In morning report the nurses told of bleeding episodes with some regularity. Our wound-ostomy NP was consulted and had tried a variety of non-adherent absorptive dressings. We had packs of Quik Clot and gel foam (hemostatic dressings) available along with a large quantity of gauze and kerlix wraps in the cabinet in his room. Don was moved to a private room near the nurse station out of concern for a roommate should he begin to hemorrhage from one of the very aggressive tumors located only centimeters from the major vessels of his neck.

Day 26, I am directed to his room as I arrive on the floor this morning. There is a gaggle of nursing staff surrounding him as he is bleeding vigorously from the tumor on the right side of his neck. He is monitoring the situation with his mirror and after several pieces of gel foam are placed on the bleeding site it begins to slow and finally stop. Dressings, which unfortunately need to be wrapped around his neck a bit snuggly to staunch the bleeding are obviously uncomfortable and a bit constricting. He can still breathe through the tracheostomy hole in his neck, if the dressing is applied with care. As the group begins to disperse he jots something on his note pad and waves me over.

So what are my chances for a larynx transplant :)? he has written. He is still fighting, using humor to diffuse the fear that he has to be feeling after another fairly significant episode of blood loss. Later that week is when he called me back to his room with the questions that he had written on his note pad that is included as the opening paragraph of this vignette. I pulled up a chair and we reviewed his concerns again. I confirmed his beliefs that his time was indeed becoming shorter, a very safe bet. The difficult question and the one that was not asked was 'how much shorter?' Because of the uncertainty of the next bleeding episode he was told that he was probably in the days to week(s) range but the bleeding could certainly start again at anytime. He had expressed concern the day before that he thought he might have to leave our unit. It was unclear why he was still harboring that concern but he was relieved to hear that he was welcome to remain with us for the duration of his journey. We spent some time in discussion about what to do with the possessions that he might still have in his apartment…if he still had an apartment. Social work was contacted to help clear up these questions and to resolve these concerns for him.

Two days later, Don was bleeding heavily again and he was reporting difficulty breathing. He was becoming anxious because he was feeling he wasn't getting any air. The movement of air through his tracheotomy seemed adequate so a trach mask delivering supplemental oxygen was applied. He was ashen pale and sweating and his respirations were shallow and rapid. A new finding on examination was significant swelling of his tongue so that it was protruding from his mouth and it too was excep-

Bradley C. Buckhout, M.D.

tionally pale. These findings suggested further progression of the tumors likely with vascular and airway compromise. He had been reluctant in the past to receive subq injection of medication but he agreed and was given lorazepam for his anxiety.

He calmed a bit but the air hunger was not relieved so a dose of morphine was provided with good relief of his distress. Don continued to try to direct his care and to maintain control of the situation which was no longer under his control. This feeling of dependence and having to rely on others for your well being is very foreign and uncomfortable for a veteran, particularly one who has lived a solitary life with little support from others. The anxiety that this creates can be an added stress which the hospice staff addresses with reassurance and caring and allowing the patient to maintain whatever sense of independence they can muster. Medications are also used to augment the non-pharmacologic interventions when needed. With these interventions Don was able to rest peacefully, his breathing unlabored and he passed away, in his sleep, as he had hoped.

Chapter 11
The Story of Juan and Jack

I would like to explore with the reader an example of comfort focused care, in contrast to the typical medical model of care delivered in an inpatient hospital, by presenting the parallel but divergent stories of two patients. Juan and Jack are both 66 year old veterans with stage IV lung cancer (which means it has metastasized to distant parts of the body from its origin in the lung). The lung cancer was due to the most common trigger, smoking and so they both have moderate COPD (chronic obstructive pulmonary disease) and both have diabetes and mild heart failure due to their heart attack in the nineties.

Juan is at home with his family, supported by a home hospice program for the last three weeks after leaving the hospital for the final time. His family doctor and the hospice team have had discussions with Juan and his family about his preferences for care now and in the future. Juan has decided that he will stay at home and use medications and oxygen and breathing treatments as he needs to but he will not go back to the hospital. He wants to have a natural death, at home with his family.

Jack is admitted to a general medical floor at the local hospital. He is worried about what is happening to him. There have been some providers who have tried to "talk him into being a DNR". He is worried that DNR means that he won't get what he needs, like nursing care or medications. He is scared by the graphic descriptions that some providers have used to describe resuscitation but he is afraid of what being a DNR would mean. He has been coughing more recently and he was sent for another chest x-ray and they drew more blood this morning but nobody has told him what they show.

Neither are eating very much but Juan has a bowl with candy, several cups with water, gatorade, a milk shake and a piece of left over pizza to nibble on. Since Jack's increased coughing was noted by speech therapy his liquids have been taken away and he can only have thickened water and red jello...always red and warm chocolate pudding.

Both are getting weaker. Juan's family helps him to get up to the bathroom and he spends most of the day in the front room in his recliner or outside on the patio in his wheelchair watching the grandkids in the pool. Jack is now flagged as a fall risk because he had difficulty standing when a nurse helped him to his wheelchair. Physical therapy saw him last week but he was not able to attend two sessions because he was short of breath so he is no longer on their schedule. He has had accidental bowel movements in bed because he couldn't get up in time and the nurses were apparently busy with someone else. The foley that was inserted when he came in through the ER is still there.

When the hospice nurse comes to check on Juan she checks his vital signs and reassures him and the family that they are what she expects them to be with the illnesses he has. She reviews his medication use and has stopped several that are no longer needed, like vitamins, medication for his cholesterol and some of his blood pressure drugs. It is stressed to him that how he is feeling is more important than the numbers. They have only checked his blood sugar once when he thought it was too low.

Jack is having his vitals checked every shift and he is having accucheks done every six hours. He has been getting small doses of insulin, 2-4 units injected before each meal time and at bedtime occasionally. He has had blood drawn at 4:30 am twice this week...he doesn't know what for, no one has told him.

Juan has oxygen at home and has tubing with nasal prongs. Sometimes when he feels short of breath he puts them in his nose and he wears it when he sleeps. He can reposition himself so he can lean forward over his bedside table to breathe. He has the fan blowing on him which also makes breathing easier. If he gets short of breath he has a nebulizer he can use. He sometimes feels smothered with the nebulizer mask so the nurse provided a mouthpiece to try. If that doesn't work small doses of morphine are available and if he gets anxious he has some lorazepam to take.

Jack also has oxygen available and every time the respiratory therapist puts the oximeter on his finger he puts the mask back on his face, which also makes him feel like he is smothering so he removes it as soon as he leaves. They have told him to leave it on because his "sats are too low" and last night they sat someone at the bedside to replace it everytime he shook it off. Unfortunately, he also couldn't spit out the mucus and he thought he would choke on the phlegm he was coughing up. The providers are concerned about opioids and benzodiazepines depressing his respiratory drive so they are very reluctant to prescribe them. When they do offer them the doses are so small they don't seem to help.

Juan's hospice interdisciplinary team meets regularly and they discuss with him and his family his concerns and recommendations for treatments going forward.

Jack is seen by a different hospitalist everyday. There is a pulmonary fellow that comes by once in a while and he has heard one of them mention the possibility of a new PET scan.

Bradley C. Buckhout, M.D.

No one seems to be in charge. What he hears is inconsistent and no one has asked him what he wants.

Juan has access to pain medications with instructions on how they are to be administered. He has a liquid version if he can't swallow the pills. He has had some episodes when his breathing became difficult, fast and shallow but after he took his morphine, relief was achieved quickly. He and his family are relieved that they have an effective way to manage these problems.

Jack also has pain and shortness of breath but the trepidation of his providers leads to inadequate dosing at intervals that are too long to be helpful and when he really needs something he sometimes has to wait 45 minutes for the nurse to bring the medication. His medications are pill or IV only. Sometimes he cannot swallow the pills and he doesn't have an IV line. He has become very anxious because of his dyspnea and the mask they strap on to deliver oxygen makes that worse.

Juan's family knows that he should have a bowel movement every other day and they keep track and make sure he is getting his liquid laxatives regularly and his hospice nurse checked him for an impaction after two days with no stool.

Jack hasn't had a bowel movement for...know one is sure how long. He has colace, a stool softener PRN for his laxative.

Juan in the last few days of his life began to collect secretions in his throat which made a disquieting rattling sound. His family positioned him on his side which largely corrected this. They were instructed on how to perform mouth care and also had an additional medication that they could use if needed. They were told by the hospice nurse what to expect as death approached and were at his side holding his hands when he took his last quiet breath.

Jack also began to have a "death rattle" but since he was flat on his back in bed with his oxygen mask strapped on his face he could not relieve it. The intern on call that evening didn't know what to do so he told the nurse that it could wait until morning. Jack passed away, afraid, struggling to breathe, alone in his hospital bed.

This comparison is unfortunately too common. The movement toward hospice and palliative care is thankfully growing. I think it is clear that it can be a wonderful alternative to the continuation of care as usual. Defining goals of care, exploring patient's understanding of their condition, a realistic appraisal of prognosis are all conversations that must be held. In short, every patient deserves honest and open communication to allow them and their loved ones to come to terms with the one universal truth, human mortality. Where do you want to spend your last days?

Bradley C. Buckhout, M.D.

Chapter 12
Mr. Gary

When one reads the essay included in the application of every prospective medical student, all are entering the calling of medicine to help people. This intent, expressed in a variety of guises, is the commitment, without which one cannot be considered a serious candidate for this career. Our most cruel failure in how we treat the sick and aged is the failure to recognize that they have priorities beyond being safe and living longer. The chance to shape one's story even in narrower and narrower confines persists. To maintain independence, even well beyond the time that it is safe and prudent is very often the overreaching goal.

This is an almost universal truth. I could give countless examples of veterans admitted to the hospital for some acute ailment that left them weaker and unable to care for themselves who were then transferred to our rehabilitation unit for "2 weeks of rehab". The very optimistic intent is for their return home, alone or with a frail and debilitated spouse to "care for them". As we meet them and explore their home situation, we frequently find an elderly person living alone with precarious, limited support from neighbors in the trailer park or a relative who stops by once in a while. It gives us pause to consider, is this a safe plan for discharge? The veteran however, is stubbornly resolved to maintain his independence for as long as possible; sometimes beyond when it is safe to do so.

My most recent example, was an admission to the CLC after a hospitalization for a small bowel obstruction. Thankfully, this 93 year old World War II veteran did not require surgery but spent several days in the intensive care unit before he recovered his gut function and could resume eating. The reason for the obstruction was not determined. Because he had undergone previous surgery for a perforated duodenal ulcer many years ago, the presumption was that the blockage developed due to adhesions in the abdomen. Mr. Gary also has a history of cancer of his esophagus which was successfully treated eight years ago. He has been living alone, in his home, here in the Valley for three years since his wife passed away. His daughters are involved, from a distance, one in California and the other in Wisconsin. Friends who have known him for four decades, reside nearby and frequently call or stop by to check on him because he has a bad habit of falling and not being able to get back up.

According to Mr. Gary he has done this 150 times, often at birthday parties and weddings but not because of excessively imbibing celebratory cocktails as one might suspect. One of his friends is a retired ICU nurse. She has been nearby on more than one of these occasions and has seen him suddenly collapse and has found him apneic and without pulse. Rather atypically, he has survived resuscitation on more than one occasion and has spontaneously revived on most. Interestingly, he has no warning that an episode is coming and often does not lose consciousness. In reviewing his medical records he has had repeated cardiac evaluations but I can find no neurology consults, no EEGs to rule out seizure activity or cataleptic drop attacks to explain these episodes. In addition to the above medical problems, he had suffered significant head trauma with a subdural hematoma ten years before in an automobile accident.

His daughters have come to stay with him at intervals to check on his welfare and to try to entice him to leave Phoenix. He steadfastly insists on staying in Arizona. They also discovered that he continues to drive his car, despite his diminishing vision, marginal hearing and these events which cause him to fall. In addition, he has a left hip that is not working well following replacement ten years ago and a frozen left shoulder due to a fall in his driveway when he dislocated that joint. Soon after he was admitted to our unit, he got out of bed without calling for assistance and tried to walk to the bathroom. He was wearing his pneumatic leg compression devices, designed to prevent blood clots. These are tethered to a pump on the foot of the bed. Unfortunately, when he reached the end of the hoses, he fell again, this time striking his head. He cut his brow but did not lose consciousness. Protocol dictated a CT scan of his head and it showed evidence of the old subdural hematoma on both halves of the brain and evidence of new bleeding in the right side where his head struck the floor.

He was transferred back to the hospital for monitoring in the ICU. While there, he was seen by the palliative care team again. They had seen him during his original admission when surgery was being contemplated to clarify what his goals of care might be. As during the first conversation, he again opted for a non-aggressive, non-surgical approach to his care. He and his daughters agreed that transfer to a neuro ICU with the possibility of neurosurgical evacuation of his hematoma was not what they wanted. They would choose palliative care and he could return to the CLC for hospice care if the bleeding into his cranial cavity continued, or to continue with the planned rehab if it did not. On his return, with family and friends at the bedside, our concern about his safety if he was alone at home was addressed. His daughters both offered to make room for him in their homes. He listened, eyes shut. When asked what he thought, he agreed that perhaps having some help around the house would be a good idea... here in Arizona.

When Caring Trumps Curing

"I have a house here, I don't owe anything on it and I don't owe any money to anyone else, I want to stay here," he said with great conviction.

We discussed that the bleeding in his head could cause him to become weak or paralyzed on one side. If that happened, he would not be able to function well enough to care for himself and may very well need hospice support. The course his body takes would become evident over the next several days to weeks and hopefully he would slowly come to accept the reality that he, like most of us, may need help at some time in our lives. It was stressed to him how lucky he was to have friends here that watch out for him and family willing to help care for him in his golden years.

For a veteran of World War II, a Black man, who has faced the challenges of growing up and raising children in America, this will require a new kind of courage that he will have to call from within. The courage to confront the reality of illness, loss of independence and his eventual mortality. The courage to seek out the truth of what is to be feared and of what is to be hoped and then the courage to act on the realization of what may come.

Unfortunately, on his return to our unit Mr. Gary seemed to share the philosophy of author Lauren Oliver, "I'd rather die my way than live yours." For those of us caring for him and his family and friends who love him, we can only hope that at some point he will have the courage, wisdom and humility to accept the help that he needs.

Bradley C. Buckhout, M.D.

Chapter 13
BILLIE

"Hey Doc how are you doing, how's the family?" greeted me as I approached Billie's bed. The nurses reported he was having chest pain again and he had been given the "Billie protocol" of medications with little change so far.

"I'm good Billie, but you're the patient, what's up? The nurse told me you're having pain again."

"She's right, I'm having that elephant on my chest thing again. It started out 9 out of 10 in intensity and then I got the 2 nitros and the 2 doses of morphine, I think those are 60 mg, right? So now the elephant is over there dancing on the ceiling and the pain is a little better."

"How much better Billie?" I inquire, knowing from previous experience that his scale is very precise.

"Well, Doc, I'd give it a 7 1/2 so I think we're making progress. I'll just keep the oxygen on a little longer and if you wouldn't mind checking back in a bit I think I'll be all right."

"Absolutely! As long as you're OK, I'll be back in half an hour."

Billie has lived here in the nursing home for nine years. He is a veteran of the Vietnam War and was saturated several times with the infamous defoliant, Agent Orange. As time has passed, the health effects of that chemical on the soldiers that were in contact with it are becoming more apparent. There is now some agreement that amyloidosis, chronic B-cell leukemias, chloracne (or similar acneform disease), diabetes mellitus type 2, Hodgkin's Disease, ischemic heart disease, multiple myeloma, non-Hodgkin's lymphoma, Parkinson's Disease, respiratory cancers, prostate cancer, peripheral neuropathies, soft tissue sarcomas all may be related to Agent Orange exposure. This is important for the veterans and their families, as compensation may be due them for these illnesses if it can be shown that they were exposed to this chemical.

Billie is 63 yrs old and is what I call the 'poster boy' for diabetic complications. If you are aware of a complication from long standing diabetes mellitus type 2, I can guarantee that Billie has it. In discussing his past with him, his family did not have a history of diabetes and although he was big, 230 pounds at six feet two inches tall he was not morbidly obese. He was diagnosed with diabetes and soon after, hypertension at age 39. Not atypically for men at that age, he did not take his conditions seriously. He continued to smoke and drink, usually took his medication but the control of his blood sugar and blood pressure were certainly not ideal. The unfortunate thing about both of these conditions is that they are silent, causing no symptoms until one day when they suddenly are not.

Billie was 43 years old when the first episode of crushing chest pain hit while he was at work. He was rushed to a local hospital and was discovered to be in the process of having a heart attack. He underwent three vessel bypass surgery at 43! His second cardiac episode was six years later and he had stents placed in four vessels. By then, he was starting to have the painful burning and numbness in his feet and lower legs, perhaps from the diabetes or that plus the effects of Agent Orange. His renal function started to decline and despite better care of his blood pressure and blood sugars, he went in to renal failure and dialysis

Bradley C. Buckhout, M.D.

started when he was 51. A diabetic foot ulcer developed slowly into osteomyelitis and after multiple surgeries he was missing his left forefoot. The wound wouldn't heal and arterial studies showed he had severe peripheral arterial disease. Angioplasty was attempted to open the vessels in his lower leg but the limb salvage was unsuccessful and he finally had a below the knee amputation of his left leg. That and dialysis ended Billie's ability to continue working. He began driver's rehab at the VA but the therapist discovered that his vision was too poor for him to drive safely and he was referred to an ophthalmologist. For those of you following along and keeping score, he of course had diabetic retinopathy and early cataracts.

He had returned home to live with his mother and his younger sister, both of whom helped him with his daily tasks. Unfortunately for Billie, his sister got married and her new husband's job was in Cleveland, so off she went. His mother, now in her late seventies was hospitalized after a fall and hip fracture and Billie needed to go somewhere while she recuperated. So at 54 years of age, he was admitted to our nursing home, initially for a two week respite stay. Billie immediately became a favorite of our staff. He was appreciative of the care that he received. He called the nurses only when he needed something and he thanked them for their help. He was always pleasant and had a smile for everyone. Billie demonstrated the oft seen curse of the nice guy…they always get the horrible diseases and complications. His mother, during her recovery from he hip fracture suffered a stroke so not only would Billie not be going home, neither would his mother. She was admitted to a community long term care facility to live out her days.

When I did return, Billie's chest pain had continued to decrease, now a 4 out of 10 so we decided that he didn't need to be sent to the hospital. This scenario repeated with some frequency over the years I cared for him, sometimes related to a meal, sometimes for no apparent reason. His chest x-rays demonstrated calcification of his coronary vessels. Cardiology had recommended no further invasive procedures but "intensive medical management" instead. On most occasions, his pain was managed with the medication combination which would slowly resolve his angina. When it failed to work, he would be transferred back to the hospital as he wanted all means utilized to keep him alive, including cardiac resuscitation.

He was transported to dialysis three times each week and for the most part, tolerated that well. He was more fatigued after each session and so he slept more. He did not have significant pain and on his non-dialysis days he did not demonstrate heart failure signs or symptoms. When he turned 60, he began to complain of pain in his right leg, different from the usual neuropathic burning. There was now a deep ache that was a little better when he let the leg hang off the edge of the bed. Vascular service was consulted again and there was evidence of arterial occlusion in the thigh and below the knee. Angioplasty was able to open the femoral artery and a stent was placed but the lower vessels were too calcified to open. After some time without an effective way to alleviate the pain of his ischemic leg, he had his second lower extremity removed. Billie took this all in stride…so to speak, and remained positive and upbeat despite all of his medical issues and the fact that he had been living in a nursing home for six years. His mental attitude and the ability to see the good in each day was an inspiration to those who had the honor to care for him. No matter what he was facing, he was always kind, appreciative and pleasant, a patient that we all enjoyed. I returned to check on him shortly after he had returned from the hospital following his second amputation and as usual his first words were, "How are you doc, how's the family?"

Bradley C. Buckhout, M.D.

"I'm doing well, Billie. How are you feeling since the surgery?"

"I'm ok Doc, the pain in my leg is gone but I have this weird feeling that I need to itch my foot...the foot that isn't there. I had some of those phantom limb feelings after the first amputation but they didn't last long, so I'm hoping it will be the same thing this time."

"I hope you are right, but if it is too annoying we could add a little dose of gabapentin for a while, that helps in some patients."

"I don't think I'll need it but thanks. By the way, could I have a plastic surgery consult?" he asked perfectly straight faced.

Surprised by this request I responded, "A plastic surgery consult? May I ask what for Billie?"

"I'd like breast implants". I couldn't tell if the twinkle in his eyes was mischievous or perhaps just the light glinting off his cataracts.

Unable to control myself I began to laugh. "Billie, why on earth do you want breast implants?"

"So I have something to play with on these long lonely nights in the nursing home," he grinned and then broke out in laughter along with me.

"Had you going there for a minute didn't I Doc?" he finally was able to get out between guffaws.

Billie entertained himself during the day watching television. His eyesight was however so poor that the standard television was too small for him to see clearly so he broke protocol in the facility and had his family purchase a large screen television that balanced on the dresser at the end of his bed. Because he was in a private room that posed no problems with bothering a roommate but because it had never been done it took, almost literally, an act of Congress to get administrative approval for this novel idea. The television was on constantly. The food network, displayed all sorts of delicacies which Billie would never be able to eat because of the dietary restrictions of diabetes, hypertension and renal failure. His response, "I can use my imagination to enjoy the recipes," was typical for his outlook and allowed him, even with all of his medical issues, to have what he considered a good quality of life.

Quality of life has become the holy grail for us all, it is the stated target to be achieved, everyone wants a "good quality of life" but what is it? What does it incorporate? The stated goal of palliative care is to maintain or improve a patient's quality of life, even in the face of greater and greater limitations being imposed by declining health and diminishing physical or perhaps mental capabilities. Even though measuring it is difficult, defining it with clarity is extremely important. Consider that medical practitioners often take "quality of life" into account when considering whether life-sustaining medical intervention should be withheld for severely disabled or ill patients. As such, coming up with a distinct definition is ethically important, and not just a case of splitting hairs.

With the life altering advances in medical care that have occurred over the last half century, extending life has become a reality. The new question, now being asked: is the goal to increase quantity of life leaving people in disabled, dependent conditions requiring institutions to care for them or should we be focused on the quality of the life being prolonged? What is quality of life? It can be defined as: "your personal satisfaction (or dissatisfaction) with

Bradley C. Buckhout, M.D.

the cultural or intellectual conditions under which you live (as distinct from material comfort)". It is, by nature, a personal definition and although there are some universal features that most would agree improve quality of life, there are others that are truly distinct and personal attributes not generalizable to the community as a whole. "Quality of life" is subjective and multidimensional, encompassing positive and negative features of life. It is a dynamic condition that responds to life events: a job loss, illness or other upheavals can change one's definition of "quality of life" rather quickly and dramatically. An analysis of scientific papers over the past 20 years shows that a precise, clear and shared definition is a long way off. Often researchers don't even attempt to define the concept, using it instead as an indicator. Among the observations made about "quality of life" is that it encompasses life satisfaction, which is subjective and may fluctuate. Multidimensional factors that include everything from physical health, psychological state, level of independence, family, education, wealth, religious beliefs, a sense of optimism, local services and transport, employment, social relationships, housing and the environment are components that play a role to varying degrees in measuring this nebulous goal for improvement. There are cultural perspectives, values, personal expectations and goals of what we want from life. It is not just the absence of disease but the presence of physical, mental and social well-being. It has been clear in the model of palliative care, that there is the need for multidisciplinary teams with different areas of training and expertise who can develop a perspective on the psychosocial and spiritual needs and not just physical/medical care for our patients.

One of the puzzles that makes defining quality of life difficult is individual interpretation of facts and events, which helps to explain how some severely disabled people can report an excellent "quality of life" while others, less debilitated can't. Part of that successful interpretation has to do with the level of acceptance of the current condition, and the ability to regulate or reject negative thoughts and emotions about that condition. Subjectivity appears to be fundamental to our understanding of "quality of life." When questions cannot be answered readily, humans have a tendency to question more and in medical fields and sociology departments this leads to research projects and if nothing else, at least a better understanding of the dilemma. This is certainly true for the "Quality of Life" conundrum. John Flanagan, an American psychologist, began work on a Quality of Life Scale in the 1970s for examining this measure in people with chronic illnesses. It has remained one of the most frequently used tools for this evaluation and can be a reliable tool for comparative measurements of a patient through his journey and also for inter-population studies. The original scoring was done based on a five point scale of the importance of the item and another five point scale on how completely the need was being met. For better separation, the satisfaction scale was eventually broadened to seven categories: delighted, pleased, mostly satisfied, mixed, mostly dissatisfied, unhappy and terrible. The scale is broken down into conceptual categories and within each of these, scale items.

Material and Physical Well Being
    Material Well Being & Financial Security
    Health & Personal Safety
    Independence, doing for yourself

Relationships with Other People
    Relations with Parents, Siblings, Other relatives
    Having & Raising Children
    Relationship with Spouse or significant other
    Relationships with Friends

Bradley C. Buckhout, M.D.

Social, Community & Civic Activities
    Activities Related to Helping & Encouraging Others
    Participation in Organizations & Public Affairs

Personal Development & Fulfillment
    Intellectual Development
    Personal Understanding
    Occupational Role
    Creativity & Personal Expression

Recreation
    Socializing
    Spectator at Recreational Activities
    Active Participant at Recreational Activities

A simpler self anchoring ladder survey tool was developed by Hadley Cantril, Princeton psychologist in his 1965 publication <u>Pattern of Human Concerns</u>. His area of research was in the new field of public opinion and he was influenced by the pioneer in the field, George Gallup who gained success in his polling techniques in the 1936 Presidential election. Cantril's Ladder is a simple visual representation of an individual's perception of their quality of life. The instructions are simple. What rung are you now standing on assuming that the bottom rung represents the worst possible life <u>for you</u>. The top rung represents the best possible life <u>for you</u>.

This "scale" of quality of life, given without further direction, allows the participant complete latitude in determining her position on the ladder, using whatever internal and external clues she chooses and the weight given to each. An extension of this research can be easily added to assess the person's view of their history, "Where were you on this ladder 5 years ago?" and also how optimistic, or contrarily how pessimistic they are about the future. "Where on this ladder do you see yourself in 5 years?" As this scale and the Flanagan QOL scale indicate, the determination of quality of life is a very personal evaluation. The determinants likely have some universality, but there are also very idiosyncratic factors that vary regionally, are different among cultures, religious groups, economic strata, educational levels and much more clearly after the 2016 Presidential campaign, political affiliations.

The OECD, Organization for Economic Cooperation & Development held their second Quality of Life Conference in October 2016. This program began in 2011 and they have created a "Better Life Index" using 11 categories and surveying 100,000 people in 180 countries around the globe.

1. Housing: conditions and spendings (e.g. real estate prices)
2. Income: household income and financial wealth
3. Jobs: earnings, job security and unemployment
4. Community: quality of social support network
5. Education: education and what you get out of it
6. Environment: quality of environmental health
7. Governance: involvement in democracy
8. Health, health care facilities and access to them
9. Life Satisfaction: level of happiness
10. Safety: murder and assault rates
11. Work-life balance

Paul Krassner, an American journalist, observed that anthropologists define happiness as having as little separation as possible between your work and your play. Their studies have shown that struggles and opportunities differ considerably dependent on the locality being surveyed. Inequities of wellbeing are widespread but the perception of what constitutes happiness and success differ considerably and what makes a Manhattan stock trader content will have little applicability to a Tanzanian shepherd.

Returning to Billie, would you be content confined to bed in a nursing home, missing both of your legs, being trundled off to dialysis three times a week? Content to watch the medical channel, history channel or the food network through eyes that are nearly blind, while being able to eat only the foods provided by the hospital kitchen and the diet Mountain Dew and pork rinds that somehow appear at your bedside? Reviewing the lists above, where would you be on the ladder today? What would enable you to move up a few rungs? Are those things within your control? Is there something that you can do to improve your relationships with people that once were meaningful in your life, is that important to you? Can you do something to improve yourself? More education, new hobbies or interests to give your life more pleasure, more meaning?

"Excellence is not a destination; it is a continuous journey that never ends." -Brian Tracy

"Self-knowledge is the beginning of self-improvement." -Baltasar Gracian

"It is not as much about who you used to be, as it is about who you choose to be." -Sanhita Baruah

"When we strive to become better than we are, everything around us becomes better too." -Paulo Coelho

Your situation now may be very dissimilar from Billie's and your answer now may be, "There is no way I could live that way," but life has a way of changing dramatically, sometimes quickly.

When Caring Trumps Curing

We have stressed repeatedly in this book the importance of planning for eventualities in the future, discussing with your spouse or children or friends, those who will likely be around and can be relied on when needed, what you would tolerate. What you would want, what you consider to be necessities for your life to be worth living. Sometimes you will have decisions to make that will be difficult, but if you have a clear image of what your Life has to be for you to be happy, those choices will be less frightening and easier to make.

Billie continued to find pleasure in his life. He spoke with his sister, in Cleveland, by phone often. Unfortunately for her, Billie would call her at 2 a.m. when he was unable to sleep and would talk to her for an hour. She visited one weekend each month and would take him to Red Lobster for a lobster dinner on those visits. It may have been one of those salt laden meals that led to another chest pain episode and admission to the hospital when we couldn't resolve his shortness of breath. A chest x-ray revealed an accumulation of fluid in the right chest between his ribs and lung. Fluid here compresses the lung tissue making less space available for delivery of oxygen to the blood. A needle was inserted between his ribs and 2500cc of clear fluid was removed and his breathing improved. Lab testing of the fluid and blood tests suggested this fluid was the result of the beginning of the end for Billie's heart. He had suffered enough damage to the muscle of his enlarged heart that it was having difficulty pumping blood around the circulatory tree, even though with the loss of his legs, it was considerably smaller than it once had been.

Congestive heart failure is a common end stage of ischemic heart disease and pleural effusions are frequently seen. Sometimes medications, specifically diuretics, can be used to reduce the fluid load but as a dialysis patient, Billie was not diuretic responsive. On occasion, his blood pressure would drop dangerously low

Bradley C. Buckhout, M.D.

when larger volumes of fluid were dialyzed from his blood. After he returned to our unit, he had recurrent bouts of shortness of breath and chest x-rays confirmed re-accumulation of the right pleural effusion. He was transported to the pulmonary lab for repeat thoracenteses and after the fourth one it was decided to leave a catheter in his chest so that it could just be attached to a suction bottle to remove the fluid rather than repeatedly sticking him. A pleurex catheter is easily tolerated with the major risk being an air leak around the tube. It may also be an access point for bacteria to enter the chest cavity. With the catheter in place, Billie began the transition to fully palliative care philosophy.

When visiting with him, "Hey, doc you been hiking lately?"

"Why, yes Billie my son and I completed another segment of the Arizona Trail this weekend, beautiful mountainous country, thanks for asking. How is your breathing doing?"

"It's a little short, I think I should be drained again."

By this point we had stopped sending him to pulmonary and we had stopped doing chest x-rays. Attaching the pleurex catheter to the suction machine and drawing off one to two liters of clear yellow fluid, based on Billie's assessment of relief was being done several times each week. These were palliative procedures, delaying the inevitable. He was able to breathe more easily after each session but the intervals between were becoming shorter and the fluid was more bloody and more tenacious making it harder to remove. It was five weeks into this process when the quantity of the fluid being removed was not sufficient to ease his breathing. We decided to get a portable chest x-ray to see why. The right side of the chest still had some fluid which appeared to be loculated, meaning it was in its own walled off space and would not be removed by the present catheter. The other problem, which had not been present before, was the appearance of fluid in the left chest too.

If we were going to continue down this path, pulmonary would need to place a second catheter in the right chest, replacing the original one and would also have to consider the addition of a catheter in his left chest as well. The pulmonologists were not in favor of this and Billie was concerned that his movements in bed would be too restricted with tubes in both sides of his chest. He called his sister and she came to town during the week so that we could all discuss the options and our plan going forward. Billie, up to this point, had requested that we do everything to prolong his life. To his sister, he had admitted that he was afraid of what dying would be like. He had a strong belief in God and did not fear what was coming after death. The process of dying was an unknown and he was having difficulty accepting its uncertainty. He was still receiving dialysis, but sessions were sometimes abbreviated because his failing heart could not sustain his blood pressure. Billie was showing signs that his body was beginning to fail in other ways. His appetite was declining, there were several full bottles of Mountain Dew and bags of Doritos, unopened and he was dozing off and on as we spoke. "Billie, I think what we are seeing are signs that your body is starting to shut down and there may not be anything that we can do to help at this point."

Wendy, taking over for Billie as he was nodding off again asked, "Doctor what do you recommend?"

"We need to discuss goals at this point. Billie has always wanted everything done to keep him alive but I'm afraid that being aggressive now will just prolong the process of dying. It is true that in medicine today there is always something more that can be done to a patient...but not always for the patient."

Bradley C. Buckhout, M.D.

Billie was back with us in the conversation. "So Doc, what do you think, what should I do?"

"Billie, I am flattered by the trust that you have in me, but this is a decision that is best made by you. I don't want to influence your decision by what I would do because your goals and your values are likely different from mine. If you would like, I can give you some potential choices to make your decision easier to make."

Both Billie and Wendy nodded their agreement.

"The hard truth is that it appears your body is finally giving up. Even if we maintain all that we are doing now we are probably looking at days to maybe at most a couple of weeks before your death. Our promise to you is that we will do whatever we can to relieve the feeling of shortness of breath that you have been having and also to medicate you for the anxiety commonly felt when you can't get your breath".

"That's reassuring to know, feeling like I'm smothering is terrifying. What about eating and dialysis?"

"At this stage in your illness, eating whatever sounds good is fine, but I've noticed that you haven't been eating much over the last several days. To continue or to stop dialysis is probably the most important question you need to consider."

"If he stops what will happen, will that make him fill up with fluid faster and maybe speed up the dying process?" asked Wendy.

"From our experience with other people who are dependent on dialysis, fading away in renal failure is actually a peaceful option. I suppose with his bad heart the fluid accumulation could make his dying a little sooner, maybe hours to days, but typically as the toxins build up in the system the patient just become more tired, sleeps longer periods and finally just dies in their sleep."

"That doesn't sound too bad. I've known the end was coming and I'm glad that you all have been honest with me. It sounds like there is no point in going back to the hospital if there is nothing more to do and maybe I should just stay here since you and the nurses all know me. I feel comfortable with your team caring for me at the end," Billie concluded.

"We all have been honored to care for you and will continue to do so to the end. Since you've made that decision, I need to ask you about your 'code status', your directions to us when your heart finally stops. As it stands, the default response is that the nurse who finds you has to call the Code Team and they will do what they have to try to restart your heart and to help you breathe. This means doing chest compressions which will break ribs, shocking your heart to try to get a rhythm back and very likely putting a tube into your windpipe to breathe for you."

"Whoa, Doc! If I'm going to die soon, why would I want all of that done to bring me back so I could die again in a few days anyway...no thanks, don't let that happen to me," Billie said without hesitation and Wendy grasping his hand nodded in agreement.

"Done. I will put an order in your chart, add a note documenting our discussion and your wishes and we will allow a natural death when the time comes. I'll give you and Wendy some time alone to discuss whether you want to continue dialysis or not and I'll be back in the morning to talk further."

The next morning with the chaplain accompanying me, we met with Billie and Wendy. They had spent the evening sharing memories of their childhood together and had concluded that there were relatives to whom Billie needed to say goodbye. They had made phone calls and the family would be arriving for the coming weekend. Once the loose ends were taken care of Billie would stop dialysis and let nature take its course.

That weekend Billie's room was full. Nieces, nephews, his brother that he had not seen for years, uncles and an elderly aunt all made the journey. They feasted on shrimp and lobster from the local Red Lobster, Billie's favorite restaurant. Billie had been an active participant in his wake. His family was able to gather and share with him their feelings and to support each other and to express what his departure will mean to the family. Not a bad arrangement and certainly more beneficial for Billie than the traditional wake when the deceased is no longer present for all of the reflections and hopefully kind words.

Over the next several days without dialysis, Billie did indeed become more short of breath. This sensation was managed with small doses of morphine with good effect. When he felt anxious, he received lorazepam and as predicted he began to sleep longer and longer periods, stopped drinking and passed away peacefully before he missed his third dialysis session. Billie was special and had endeared himself to the entire VA community. The family requested a memorial service in the hospital chapel the following week. The family filled one pew but the rest of the benches were filled with hospital and nursing home staff there to say their farewell. A large photo of Billie with several flower arrangements adorned the altar and Father Matt presided over the service. At the completion of his prepared eulogy and prayers he asked if anyone in the assemblage had any remembrances to share about Billie. A story or experience to give a picture of who he was in life, how he influenced or touched us when he was here.

Silence...nothing. Seconds extended to half a minute, the silence was becoming uncomfortable. Should I tell my favorite Billie story in the chapel, at his memorial? I stood up. "Well, I've got a story. One day several months ago Billie called me to his bedside and asked me for a plastic surgery consult...." This story had the congregation laughing and started a flood of similar happy recollections, a fitting end to a special veteran's life.

The End of Life is Universal. The when can usually not be controlled but the HOW often can be, especially when brought on by chronic illnesses which take the spark away slowly...dying can be done well, or very badly and it is in many cases YOUR choice. Billie had taken control of how his life would end and on his terms conducted what we and his family would call a "good" death. A positive experience without the suffering, stress and drama that can be a part of the final act.

Bradley C. Buckhout, M.D.

Chapter 14
Gratitude, Forgiveness, Apology, Love

Palliative care seeks to address the spiritual and psychological challenges that face each patient as their life draws to a close. There has been much research done to address the impact that unresolved conflict or remorse, or in simple terms, lack of resolution or closure has on the last days of a person's existence. The amount of psychological baggage and subconscious distress a person is bearing can contribute to physical suffering, insomnia, anxiety, loss of hope and despair. Techniques for resolving these sometimes unstated or unrecognized needs are often very powerful and operate on several levels. When reviewing the major religious philosophies and the rituals to be completed as death approaches there is more in common than one would initially think. Much of the focus, for the patient as well as the family, is seeking the peace of forgiveness and redemption in preparation for departing this life and entering whatever comes next.

Hospice psychologists often incorporate the Four Questions to open a dialogue and to focus attention on these unmet needs. The questions are simple, but often open long closed portals.

1. Is there anyone you would like to thank?

2. Is there anyone you would like to forgive?

3. Is there anyone to whom you want to apologize?

4. Is there anyone to whom you want to express your love?

When Caring Trumps Curing

Four simple questions; but the power they provide for resolving old losses, old conflicts and for expressing gratitude and love often open the path to healing old wounds. With the release of the negative emotions, associated physical symptoms can be managed more easily. The next step, after identifying the person or persons that need to hear these words, is for the patient to dictate a letter expressing their feelings. The therapeutic benefit for the patient is likely just the framing of the thoughts, but if the letter is actually sent it may help the healing of the other half of the damaged relationship or further bolster one that was already healthy. I have witnessed a woman dying of cancer and struggling to breathe. When she was asked the four questions and started to compose her thoughts to her daughter for whom she was offering forgiveness there was a visible easing, almost immediately, of her distressed breathing, a relaxation of her shoulders which had been unconsciously drawn up to her ears due to the internal tension and distress she was harboring. What is the mechanism of this response? Is it due to a change in neurochemistry, a change in perception or as some cultures, religions and philosophers believe a change in something greater than the self?

Cultures of South Pacific Islanders and Hawaii have a philosophy of disease and origins of suffering based on the commission of errors, anger or misconduct. Secrecy gives the power to the misdeed and until it is confessed the illness will not be relieved. A Hawaiian healing practice of reconciliation and forgiveness, the name of which translates into English simply as 'correction' is used for those with serious illness. In this practice, if one would take complete responsibility for one's life, then everything one sees, hears, tastes, touches, or in any way experiences would be one's responsibility because it is in one's life. The problem would not be with our external reality, it would be with ourselves. Total Responsibility, according to philosopher Hew Len, advocates that everything exists as a projection from inside the self. The

Bradley C. Buckhout, M.D.

secret is, there is no such thing as "out there," everything happens to you in your mind. Everything you see, everything you hear, every person you meet, you experience in your mind. You only think it's "out there" and you think that absolves you of responsibility. In fact it's quite the opposite: you are responsible for everything you think, and everything that comes to your attention.

Forgiveness has a powerful quality of healing and transformation that can promote the release of life's deepest fears. These fears come from feelings, ideas and attitudes that are projected on to others and objects in our consciousness. These projections are the externalizations of guilt and blame toward others. These negative projections are a defense against anxiety and fear. Forgiveness is the energy that releases these outwardly directed projections. A sincere statement "please forgive me" offered up to the Universe is sufficient. But this request can also be directed to a person or persons from whom you are asking forgiveness. In my practice this has been a common situation. Many of our veterans returned from conflicts and alienated family and friends due to their inability to assimilate back into civilian life. Perhaps they were abusing alcohol or other substances, couldn't hold a job and dropped out of society. For many reasons they have lost touch. Some seek resolution of these issues as their life winds down. In the Four Question technique the direction of this step is reversed, is there anyone you would like to forgive, rather than the statement, please forgive me. Carrying resentment to the grave resolves nothing and forgiveness at this stage in life may help unburden the patient and perhaps ease the mind of the one who has been resented for so long. At the end of life, it is required that everything to which we are connected in this world is left behind. Forgiveness is a tool that helps release the negative attachments that have been built throughout life as the patient proceeds through the dying process.

When Caring Trumps Curing

Gratitude is a powerful energy that can open the heart. Saying "thank you," with sincerity, is healing and it doesn't really matter who or what you're thanking. Thank your body for all it does for you, even though it is now failing. Thank yourself for being the best you can be. Thank God. Thank the Universe. Specifically thank people who have helped you on your journey. Thank those who have made you the person you have become, those who encouraged and supported you, those who have helped you overcome the obstacles in your life. Gratitude alters how the world is viewed and is available to provide for a fuller, more conscious and deliberate expression of the self. Gratitude changes the perception of life events and allows seeing, feeling and experiencing with depth, clarity and understanding each person, event or expression. The practice of gratitude both grounds us and opens within us a greater awareness that touches the infinite beyond.

Appreciation opens the doorway to present moment awareness. It has been expressed in many philosophies that to gain internal peace one must live in the present and be fully aware of the now. There is both awareness of the outer world as well as the inner self simultaneously. Awareness is the opening to the expanded world and its many dimensions. This expansion is the source of power of appreciation because it eliminates judgment or preconception from the truth of reality.

Kindness is basically a means of acceptance that holds that whatever the person, circumstance or condition, the kind response is one without judgment or a projection of superiority. The action of kindness comes from the insight that everyone is battling something that you know nothing about.
The response; be kind always, will serve well and assist in the preparation for the transition that follows death.

Bradley C. Buckhout, M.D.

You are responsible for everything in your mind, even if it seems to be "out there." This realization can be painful, and difficult to accept. To begin to adopt this philosophy, choose something that you already know you've caused for yourself. Are you over-weight, addicted to nicotine, alcohol or some other substance? Do you have anger issues? Do you have someone to whom you need to apologize for some past behavior? Start there and say you're sorry. That's the whole step: I'm sorry. There is more power if you say it more clearly: "I realize that I am responsible for the (issue) in my life and I feel terrible remorse that something in my consciousness has caused this."

Say "I Love You". Tell the people that you cherish, those people that have meant the most to you during your life. Don't assume they know, tell them. It is important, soon you won't be here and if they are important to you, they need to know, now. If you are religious, say it to your God. Each of us will face our death alone. Others may support and help us in the final process of our dying with comfort and prayers, but it will be the practices of life and the ability to apply those practices during the dying process that will lead to the peace and grace sought as the journey continues.

Chapter 15
PASTOR JEFFERSON AND BROTHER WILL

Religious and spiritual issues at the end of life can have a very strong influence on the course of care in the last days of life. Hopefully, the powerful positive influence of faith will reduce the anxiety of what will come after this existence. Belief in coming redemption, an eternal idyllic existence and the end of the suffering are promised to those who believe. Meeting the Father for reconciliation, reincarnation as a higher form, depending on the religious doctrine that one follows will be a comfort in the coming transition. In contrast to those positive images are the fears of retribution, the unknown, the uncertainty of what will happen when the eyes close for the last time.

Palliative care teams are multidisciplinary and have chaplain services available. The chaplain can professionally assist with resolving conflicts and supporting the religious practices and preferences of a diverse range of spiritual beliefs. They are a great comfort to those willing to accept their counsel and guidance. The chaplain is rarely the first member of the team to have contact with a patient, so during the initial meetings, a palliative care team member will ascertain the patient's and his/her family's spiritual/religious/existential beliefs, practices, preferences and needs. This is often referred to as taking a spiritual history.

Faith - Do you consider yourself a spiritual person?
Importance - Is faith important to you?
Community - Are you part of a spiritual or faith community?

Bradley C. Buckhout, M.D.

Address - How can we address these issues and respect your beliefs in your care?

Offering these questions, as part of the routine medical history taking, normalizes and gives equal validity to them and opens the door for further conversation and exploration. This may not be the area of expertise of the nurse practitioner or physician but for more in depth discussion the chaplain can be consulted.

The longer I've been in medicine, the more I have learned to suppress the self doubt of uncertainty. Patients remain mysteries. There are unanswerable questions, unexpected results, some who survive longer than expected and others who succumb suddenly. This uncertainty applies also to the spiritual sphere... there are questions that cannot be answered. But with supportive discussions, patients will often come to their own realization and resolutions without the doctor having to "fix" a problem. Palliative care, by its nature, tends to work within the confines of unsolvable situations and through creative thinking and a dedicated focus on improvement will make the untenable situation less so. Comfort for the patient and family physically, emotionally and spiritually are the ultimate goals for the team. Occasionally, rigidly held beliefs make this goal almost unattainable. We have encountered families whose faith created, what to us appeared to be, unnecessary and unneeded suffering. Restrictions on what we would normally do to achieve comfort were rejected out of an unshakeable belief system alien to our role in improving the last days for our patient. These patients, although competent in a legal sense and therefore capable of choosing their course of treatment, chose to avoid interventions that could have perhaps lengthened their life in one case and could have made the existence of the other much less of an ordeal for all involved.

When Caring Trumps Curing

Pastor Jefferson was an elder in his Evangelical Christian Church. He had been born in the South, in a fundamentalist denomination with very strict Biblical interpretations. When he moved to Arizona thirty years ago, he founded a congregation of like-minded souls and had nurtured his parishioners for three decades. This was a poor church and he devoted his time to caring for its members and not so much to caring for himself. He began to lose weight, initially not a bad thing as he had let himself get excessively heavy which made getting around in the heat of the Valley of the Sun a sweat soaked challenge. Even with his loss of weight, he began to notice walking was becoming painful. His legs would ache after 3 blocks, a few months later 2 blocks and eventually just walking from the parking lot to his office in the rectory would make his legs cramp. Thankfully, a few minutes of rest would relieve this pain and he could go on about his business.

Prayers for answers and relief weren't resolving the problem, but sometimes changes are small and maybe he just wasn't seeing it clearly yet. Maybe he wasn't worthy of the Lord's intervention. When he was in the Army infantry, he had not practiced the tenets of his faith. He had killed. He had taken the Lord's name in vain. He had mistreated his body. He continued his ministry with increased vigor and paid little attention to the numbness in his feet and lower legs. One day, when he took off his socks, he noticed the big toe on his left foot was black…blacker than the rest of his foot and there was a smell that he recognized. The smell that one never forgets. He had first encountered it in Vietnam when his platoon, on the tail of a Vietcong sapper squad, entered a village in the jungle and discovered the bloated bodies of dozens of villagers who had been slain probably two days before…the smell of dead flesh. His response, unfortunately not uncommon for men in general and veterans in particular, was to wash his foot, spray it with Bactine and to ignore it. It wasn't until two weeks later, after the toes of his right foot had become black and a hole in his left ankle appeared when a black leathery scab came off that his wife persuaded him to come to the emergency room. He was admitted to the hospital and was seen first by the medicine team as his blood sugar was 436 and his white blood cell count was 23,000. Podiatry was also consulted. This unfortunately, is a very common scenario. Poorly controlled diabetes leading to neuropathy and then a diabetic foot ulcer, bone infection and then amputation of the non-viable tissue. There was visible evidence that the damaged tissue extended above the ankle, out of the realm of the podiatrist's expertise and so vascular surgery also saw him. They recommended angiograms, injecting dye into the arteries to decide at what level the blood vessels were blocked. The lower legs did not appear to be salvageable, the damage was so severe, gangrene had set in and amputation probably below the knees on both sides would be needed to save Pastor Jefferson's life.

He refused. He refused the angiograms. He refused the proposed surgery. He refused insulin. He took antibiotics for a while but was not interested in any alteration in his body and amputation was certainly not going to be performed. He was not delirious, he was capable of understanding the consequences of his choices and his wife supported his decision. The distress this caused the medicine team and the surgeons led to an ethics consult as this patient was, in their minds, not thinking clearly and should not be able to make the choice to die when there was clearly a solution that would prevent it.

The ethics committee is a diverse group of volunteers within the hospital, made up of physicians, social workers, psychologists, clergy and lay people. One of the overriding principles in all ethics deliberations is the preservation of patient autonomy. It was very clear that despite the discomfort felt by the medical providers and the knowledge that their advice was medically prudent, Pastor Jefferson was the one responsible for his life. A patient has the right to make decisions, even decisions that others would not choose, even if those decisions are responsible for suffering and potentially shortening his life. In the bigger context, many of our patients are admitted to the hospital in dire straights because of those autonomous decisions. The ethics committee's opinion supported Pastor Jefferson's decision based on that autonomy principle and he was then transferred to our unit for the stated reason of rehab and strengthening so he could return home. The fallacy of that plan was evident upon our first meeting. There was no way, without Divine intervention, that he was ever going to be able to stand again and walking was a total impossibility. Approaching his room from the nurses' station, there was an odor escaping from under his closed door. The odor that is familiar to providers dealing with necrotic tissue, a pungent, somewhat sweet, acidic smell that cannot be mistaken for anything else. Opening the door bathed us in the stench, but he and his wife were quietly conversing apparently oblivious to the overwhelming smell of dying flesh.

We began by exploring the purpose of the Pastor's transfer to our unit. They replied that he was here to get stronger, to be able to transfer to a wheelchair so he could go home. He had not been able to walk for some weeks now and he was a very thin, ill appearing man with muscular wasting of his face giving him a hauntingly skeletal appearance. His ribs were easily counted and his abdomen was sunken. His limbs were dark sticks with little remaining muscle. Each of his legs was swaddled in bulky white bandages with some orange-red staining suggesting the podiatry service was still involved in his care. After asking his permission, we, with some trepidation, began to unwrap his feet. Dressing removal with extensive wounds is often painful, so before proceeding very far we asked, "Pastor, would you like some

Bradley C. Buckhout, M.D.

medication for pain before we get too far along in removing the dressings?"

"No, thank you. I will not be needing any medication for this process, proceed."

We began unwrapping layer after layer of dressing and discovered the expected betadine soaked gauze pads applied to the wounds. Betadine is an antiseptic and tends to dry wounds and reduces bacterial growth. It is frequently used to stabilize and clean up wounds with much necrosis like we had been warned we would find here. All of the toes on both feet were black, the fifth toe on the left was still attached only by a thin strip of fibrous debris and it came off when the dressing was removed. The tendons on the lateral ankle were exposed, a glistening white strand running the length of the wound, partially shrouded in a soupy tan mucousy liquid. There was also a large piece of flesh missing from the ball of the foot with evidence of bone appearing at the base of the second and third toes. The right had fared little better with the majority of the tip of the right great toe missing. The tendons of the top of the right foot were exposed, but there were pieces of dry black eschar adherent in places and some places where it was easily picked off with a forceps. The right heel was also involved, it was capped by a black eschar that was loose around the edges and had a gray slimy looking material in the cracks. Both lower legs to about mid calf were darker than the skin above and were swollen and reddened. The Pastor very stoically endured all of the dressing removal and his wife's face remained impassive. One of the students with me left the room to avoid fainting.

"After seeing these wounds for the first time, what can we do to help you? I understand that you have told the surgeons you don't want them to remove the dead tissue."

When Caring Trumps Curing

"That's right, I just want to get stronger so that we can go home. I have things that I need to do there," he replied.

"I hope you can do that as well. But I worry with what we are seeing in your legs and feet that you may not be able to get better and that you actually could get much worse and may die. I wonder if you've given any thought to what you will do or what you will let us do if you don't show signs of improvement?" I offered trying to see if there were alternatives he had considered.

"I am going to get better, it is not your responsibility. It is in His hands and I trust that with the prayers of my church, if I am worthy I will be healed," he replied with confidence.

"Can you help me understand your beliefs? You are obviously a man with very strong faith in a Divine power but does that prevent you from accepting the care of those who are trying to help you achieve your work?"

"Nothing happens that God does not ordain, cause, or allow. We are constantly surrounded by Divine intervention, even when we are ignorant of it or blind to it. We will never know all of the times and all of the ways God intervenes in our lives. Divine intervention can come in the form of a miracle, such as a healing," he responded with more fervor in his voice, almost as if he were in his pulpit.

"I understand but could your medical providers not be the instruments of the Divine will?" I pursued.

"I am imperfect, as we all are and I believe that the trials of the flesh which I have been sent to endure are an atonement, a test of my faith and if I prove worthy a healing will occur."

Bradley C. Buckhout, M.D.

With a better understanding of his firmly held beliefs, our approach, as with all of our patients, was to attempt to align what skills we had with his goals and what he would permit. He remained a patient on our unit for several weeks. He would allow debridement of his wounds which reduced some of the malodor from the room but was clearly insufficient to allow healing. He remained pleasant and reserved. He did not allow us to provide antibiotics but neither did the swelling or redness progress in his legs. He was not febrile and never developed signs that he was becoming systemically ill, perhaps evidence in itself of a small miracle. He also would not receive pain medications, despite what in my experience with countless other patients should have been what we in medicine euphemistically call extreme discomfort. His wounds would not allow him to bear weight on his legs. He spent all of his time in bed and we had attempted to get him into a wheelchair using our ceiling lift on the only three occasions that he would allow.

Questions to him and his wife on how they expected to get him in and out of bed or to the bathroom at home without a lift were answered simply with, "We'll manage."

We offered to have visiting nurse services come to their home to assist them and they declined choosing instead to rely on the members of their church to aid his return. Then one day, with no apparent change in his condition, he declared he was ready to be discharged to return to his home and his ministry. His wife and some elders of his church arrived and spirited him off our unit in a wheelchair to a waiting church van parked out front. We did not see him again. I don't know the details of what happened after he left. Was our view as medical professionals correct, did he succumb to the ravages of his ischemic lower extremities and diabetes and die of an overwhelming infection? Or were his faith and beliefs strong enough to sustain him through this ordeal?

When Caring Trumps Curing

There are so many intangible factors that effect a patient's course. Faith and beliefs are not inconsequential in their contributions to the direction that an illness will take. The strength of support from a close family, which may include a faith community and friends, with prayers and an emotional boost can sustain many through very difficult times. There have been cases who have appeared near the end of life, who were apparently revived by the arrival of distant family, perhaps pulled from the brink by the positive energy and well wishes. It is also true that despite these forces, patients still succumb to their diseases. Sometimes later but inevitably, they arrive at their final destination.

Observationally, certainly not based on scientific evidence, there appears in some patients, an ability to determine the moment of their death, some control of when they finally let go. We have seen this in several forms. There is a distant relative who is coming to say her last goodbyes. We have alerted her that time is growing short (within the fallible precision of our prognostication skill) and she will be here soon. Knowing this fact, even when minimally responsive, has kept patients going until the last meeting is concluded. It is also true that close, hovering families can sometimes hold their loved one in a position somewhere between life and death. There is always someone at the bedside, trying to comfort, speaking softly, singing, stroking the hair, offering nourishment...anything to help. They fear leaving because someone must be there, he can never be alone. "We don't want him to die alone, we need to be with him," they say with absolute conviction. The patient hangs on, sometimes with retained ability to communicate other times apparently somnolent and unresponsive. What we have experienced repeatedly, after days or weeks of this constant vigil, the patient finds an opening through which to finally escape when the family member steps out of the room to make a phone call or to grab a bite to eat. Perhaps they don't want an audience, perhaps they don't want to

Bradley C. Buckhout, M.D.

leave with a family member clasping their hand, they depart when they are alone. Some families are dismayed and feel guilty but we reassure them that we see this frequently and in many cases have prepared them in advance. We suggest that giving the patient permission, verbally and even by departing briefly, will on occasion allow this journey, which may have been long and difficult, to finally come to an end. Families who have prepared emotionally for this final step accept our suggestion, others unfortunately have a very difficult time letting go.

Brother Will was a middle aged African-American veteran who had been discovered, while in the hospital, to have an inoperable biliary tree cancer. These tumors are not common and often present with jaundice due to blockage of the bile ducts, causing bile to back up in the blood. He had nausea, bloating and abdominal pain and a tube had been inserted through his flank into his gallbladder to drain the bile externally. His immediate family, an elderly mother and his three sisters were at his bedside when I first met them as part of an ethics consult. The ethical question revolved around the request to place a feeding tube. Will's ability to make decisions had been questioned by his family. His sisters were the ones pushing to have a tube placed and they felt he could not decide to refuse it.

Will had suffered a stroke eight months earlier, which resulted in expressive aphasia. For those not medically trained, the stroke damaged the part of the brain responsible for producing coherent thought and speech. In response, Will and many other stroke victims find speaking so frustrating that they become mute rather than produce the meaningless jumble of words when they try to communicate.

This family was very close and were also strongly religious. The sisters were a gospel singing group who had recorded and also toured across the country performing with Will, as their manager, up until his stroke. Will's wife had passed away some years before but he had not changed his will and had not completed advanced directives. By default, his mother would become his surrogate decision maker, but it was clear at her advanced age, that dementia had robbed her of her ability to provide meaningful input. Next in line for surrogacy were his sisters. They spoke in unanimity, which simplified the debate somewhat. Had there been a dispute among them, it would have added another layer of complexity to the resolution of the issue.

Earlier in the hospital stay, a nasogastric feeding tube had been placed, with some difficulty. Will had suffered a bloody nose that had been difficult to stop due to the blood thinners being used to reduce his risk of developing blood clots in his legs and to prevent a new stroke. His stroke was the first manifestation of previously unidentified atrial fibrillation and he had stayed on his warfarin since then. The tube feedings caused some bloating and Will had vomited and developed an aspiration pneumonitis following that episode. That landed him in the ICU for several days, but thankfully didn't require intubation and ventilator support for his breathing. Shortly after he returned to the regular hospital floor he had pulled out his feeding tube. When he was approached by the nurse with another, he emphatically shook his head and with remarkable clarity said "NO!"

His sisters, not wanting to give up on their brother requested that he be restrained so the tube could be replaced. The staff declined. The sisters then requested a PEG tube be placed, surmising that it would be less annoying but not considering the risks of its insertion or maintenance thereafter. The gastroenterologists who were involved in the case did not feel that the tube was indicated as Will could still eat if he chose to. General surgery declined tube placement as he had cancer and was too high a surgical risk. Interventional radiology was then consulted and they agreed that placement of the PEG was possible if Will agreed. The inpatient service was in a quandary, there was apparent disagreement between the patient and the family and there remained some question about Will's ability to comprehend the decision he was being asked to make. It was fairly clear that he did not want the nasogastric tube replaced and had also shaken his head indicating "no" when they presented the idea about placing another tube through his abdominal wall.

Mental health had been consulted and they opined that despite his verbal limitations he was apparently aware of the consequences and implications of his decisions, the definition of capacity. The concept of preservation of autonomy for patients has been presented several times throughout this work. A corollary to the basic foundation established by the Bill of Rights is the common-law principle of self-determination that guarantees the individual's right to privacy and protection against the actions of others that may threaten bodily integrity. An extension of self-determination includes the right to exercise control over one's body, for example, the right to accept or refuse medical treatment. It is expected that when one freely accepts or refuses treatment, he or she is competent to do so, and is, therefore, accountable for the choices made. However, concerns naturally arise when an individual is deemed to be incompetent. How then is he protected from poor decisions? An individual determined to be incompetent can no longer exercise the right to accept or refuse treatment and a surrogate decision maker must assume that role.

To refresh the reader's memory, the terms capacity and competency both deal with the patient's ability to maintain control over their lives and whether they are able to do so or not. Competency is court determined, based on the preponderance of evidence presented to a judge. Medical opinion is certainly incorporated but may not be the exclusive information garnered. Competency is a legal term referring to individual "having sufficient ability... possessing the requisite natural or legal qualifications" to engage in a given endeavor. This is a broad concept encompassing many legally recognized activities, such as the ability to enter into a contract, to prepare a will, to stand trial and for our purposes, to make medical decisions. The definition, therefore, must be clarified depending on the issue in question. Simply put, competency refers to the mental ability and cognitive capabilities required to execute a legally recognized act rationally. After determining that the de jure incompetent cannot make prudent decisions in his or her own best interest, the court will assign a guardian to make decisions on the person's behalf.

Capacity is determined by a physician, often (although not exclusively) by a psychiatrist, and not the court. Capacity refers to an assessment of the individual's cognitive abilities to understand, appreciate, and manipulate information and form rational decisions. The patient evaluated by a physician to lack capacity to make reasoned medical decisions is referred to as de facto incompetent, i.e., incompetent in fact, but not determined to be so by legal procedures. Such individuals cannot exercise the right to choose or refuse treatment, and they require another individual, a surrogate, to make decisions on their behalf. Protection of the physician naturally arises when an individual freely chooses a course of treatment rationally and with full knowledge of the potential consequences and untoward events. It is not surprising that the frequent requests for psychiatric consultation in matters of competency are often based on the physicians' perceived need to "cover themselves" from a medical-legal perspective. The physician is not automatically authorized to perform medical treatment on the behalf of a patient deemed incapable of making

Bradley C. Buckhout, M.D.

reasoned medical decisions. Similarly, a physician who withholds treatment from an incompetent patient who refused treatment could be liable for any untoward events that occurred to the patient if that physician had not taken reasonable steps to obtain some other legally valid authorization for treatment. Thus, when carefully explored and appropriately employed, the capacity assessment serves to protect the physician rendering treatment as well as the patient.

The ethics consultation team supported Brother Will's refusal of a feeding tube and so the inpatient service requested he be transferred to our CLC hospice unit for continuation of his care. Prior to their arrival, we had already had several conversations but the sisters had not come to the realization that there was little more medically that could be done for their brother. It was their belief that if he was better hydrated he would regain his appetite and his strength and be able to get out of bed. Will unfortunately, was also paralyzed on his right side due to the stroke so was impaired functionally even prior to this hospitalization. He had seen oncology prior to his transfer but due to his liver dysfunction and his poor performance status he was not felt to be a chemotherapy candidate.

The gospel sisters pressed the feeding tube again on our first meeting in the CLC. After a lengthy discussion, it was decided they would try to feed him by hand, a plan that Will would not enjoy. They proposed, or more accurately demanded that he receive continued intravenous feedings. After some lengthy explanations it was eventually accepted by the sisters that parenteral nutrition (nutritive fluids given through a vein) tended to do a better job feeding the tumor, not the patient. It is also associated with potentially lethal blood infections and was not designed for long term nutritional support. They acquiesced with

When Caring Trumps Curing

some reluctance, but had a fall back position, IV fluids. I felt that we had accomplished significant progress moving to this more reasonable position. Part of the challenge of treating palliative and hospice patients is that the provider is also treating the family. There are often very complicated dynamics, known only to the family members that will color the interactions with the provider. It is very clear that agreeing to some of the family requests that have little potential for harm, but with limits established at the beginning, can make the provider an ally rather than an adversary.

It was agreed that we would give Will intravenous fluids, as long as there was evidence of improvement and there was no evidence that we were doing harm. The next challenge was to define what benefit they were hoping to see. Their goals were modest. They hoped he would be able to eat more and be able to sit on the side of the bed. Fluids were started at only two ounces an hour, slow enough that we shouldn't cause harm, but fast enough to meet the needs of the family. We continued for six days with no appreciable change in his nutritional intake. He continued to resist their efforts at feedings, turning his head away and clenching his mouth shut. It was apparent that Will was not interested in living as long as possible, nor living as long as his sisters wanted. He was tired. After the first week of fluids, his lower legs started to swell and he developed a cough. Listening to his chest, I could hear evidence that he was beginning to accumulate fluid in his lungs. I met with his sisters and expressed my concern and my observations. Will was not getting better, he was showing no interest in eating and had not been able to sit up. We were beginning to cause harm with the IV fluids, it was time to stop. I acknowledged their love for their brother and that it was very hard to realize that his time was becoming short. We discussed that there was nothing left to be done to alter the course of his disease and I asked them to stop making his eating a contentious

Bradley C. Buckhout, M.D.

battle between them. Sometimes, I said, love is just being there and letting go. Tearfully, they agreed and they began to call the family together to say goodbye.

It was only a few days after the fluids stopped that Will slipped into unconsciousness, his eyes a bright golden hue from his severely elevated bilirubin. Then one morning the nurse came to the desk, "He's gone," she told me. "The family is at the bedside." I entered the room. The three sisters were there, tears were flowing and a nephew that I had not met was there as well, speaking to his uncle in obvious distress, "No, no, you can't go, please Uncle Will!" When he heard me he stepped aside and I placed my stethoscope on Will's chest and listened intently for a full minute. There were no sounds, no cardiac tones, no respirations and as I listened I watched his face. His golden eyes were partially open, unseeing, unmoving. Will had passed away, peacefully, surrounded by his family.

I offered my condolences, had a few words with the sisters and went to the computer to document his passing. Shortly after I sat down the nurse returned. "They think he is breathing again, they want you to come back and check him," she said shaking her head. I returned to his room, the looks of hopeful anticipation melted away after I repeated my previous examination with the same result. "I'm sorry folks, Will is gone," I said. The nephew began to weep. I turned to him and asked, "Your whole family has very strong religious beliefs. If the scriptures are correct, is he not going to a much better place? Is there not some cause for relief that he is free of the suffering from the cancer?"

"You are right, I know those things but the flesh is weak, it is hard to give him up, but thank you for the reassuring reminder."

When Caring Trumps Curing

I have been practicing medicine for almost forty years, in training, private practice as a family doctor and now in a skilled nursing facility with patients facing very complicated and potentially life threatening illness. Medicine, as it is currently practiced has become very much more technologically dependent. The capabilities of what can be measured, imaged, monitored and explained has radically expanded. Science has progressed, unravelling the human genome to search for patient specific treatments, biologic chemotherapy agents that are built specifically for the genetics of a patient's individual cancer. These developments are so incredible that a few short years ago they would have been found only in a science fiction novel. Despite the power of these tools there are still many patients whose response to therapy, or disease course, or symptoms are simply unexplainable. I have been seeing patients for four decades and despite the variety of that experience, I am still seeing things on nearly a weekly basis that I have never previously encountered. One would think that after so many years, uncertainty would be a rarity, but it is actually a fairly constant companion.

One of the hallmarks of a good family practitioner, a specialty whose challenge is in its breadth, is the realization that a patient's situation is beyond the scope of one's experience or skill. There is a sense that the patient is not reacting as expected, I have reassessed my assumptions, reviewed my differential diagnosis and reevaluated the treatment plan and there is something I am not seeing...time to call a specialist colleague. But this is also where the art of medicine is most important. Patients and families don't expect physicians to have all the answers, but they do expect them to care.

The time I have spent sitting at the bedside of a patient allowing them to tell their story, to share with me who they are and what their aspirations and goals are is often far more instructive and

Bradley C. Buckhout, M.D.

therapeutic than another battery of tests or scans. Listening, a vital part of the art of medicine cannot be replaced by the latest technologic advance. Palliative & hospice medicine is a modern specialty that utilizes the time honored traditions of personal contact, empathy, support for the patient and family at a time in a patient's life When Caring Trumps Curing.

Appendix A

The Veterans Administration has developed a program titled the Life Sustaining Treatment Decision Initiative. The target population for this discussion are veterans with significant chronic medical conditions that may lead to death in the next two years if they progress in the usual fashion. This progress note, which is entered in the electronic medical record, will be durable across all locations within the VA whether it is completed in an outpatient clinic, the hospital, during a community living center admission or during a home based primary care visit. It includes the patient's wishes for resuscitation attempts (the typically entered "full code" or "DNR" order) but goes much further. There is an assessment by the provider as to the competency of the patient to make these decisions, a notation of the surrogate decision maker and then questions about the veteran's goals and his desires for a variety of medical interventions. There is much more opportunity for including explanations and qualifiers than in the previous advanced directive documents that are frequently found in the medical record with the qualifier "it would depend" without further explanation when attempting to address some life and death medical decisions.

LSTDI
The Life Sustaining Treatment Decision Initiative is a product of the National Center for Ethics in Healthcare. This organization provides study and guidance for ethical care of the veteran population in the VA system, the largest integrated health network in the country. The goal of this initiative is to assist veterans in defining their goals for their life as well as healthcare and then providing support for achieving them. The starting point for this important step is the Goals of Care Conversation.

Bradley C. Buckhout, M.D.

At present, this is most often carried out in the hospital, when some critical illness requires urgent life or death decisions initiated by a medical provider trained in the techniques of this sometimes emotional discussion. The vision for the program is that these conversations will eventually be introduced by a patient's own provider, in an office visit, under much less stressful conditions with time for reflection and deliberation.

Who are the patients for which an LSTD discussion should be completed? There are many triggering events or changes in condition that make this appropriate:

1. After admission to a VA community living center. These are skilled nursing facilities and often accept very medically complex, debilitated patients.
2. At a primary care visit (including home based primary care) within 6 months after the patient comes under the care and is identified as a high risk patient, or at the earliest opportunity if the patient has an expected survival of 6 months or less.
3. After a new palliative care consultation. This team is consulted when a patient has a symptom burden that is making life difficult or is facing conditions that may shorten his life dramatically.
4. Prior to referral to hospice. This makes perfect sense. If the patient's disease has led to a condition that could make death within the next few months a likely possibility, discussion about his wishes for resuscitation and other life supporting measures and a frank discussion of goals to make the remaining days as meaningful and pleasant as possible.
5. Prior to initiating or discontinuing a treatment intended to prolong the patient's life when the patient would be expected to die soon without the treatment.
6. After admission to a VA acute care hospital.
7. Prior to a procedure involving general anesthesia, initiation of hemodialysis, cardiac catheterization, electrophysiology studies

or any procedure that poses a high risk of serious arrhythmia or cardiopulmonary arrest. This raises an interesting dilemma. Most surgeons will insist on temporary suspension of a DNR order in the immediate (30 day) post-operative period. The reasoning has been explained that for a patient to agree to the surgical procedure, there must be an intent on getting better, to improve and that all efforts should be expended to save a patient who has expressed this wish. So, before you undergo a surgery discuss this policy with your surgical team.

8. Prior to writing Do Not Attempt Resuscitation/Do Not Resuscitate orders or other orders to limit life sustaining treatments, including POLST or similar orders.

9. At any patient encounter when the patient (or surrogate) expresses a desire to make decisions about limiting or not limiting LSTs in the patient's current treatment plan.

In many situations, this discussion may occur over a series of visits and the document completed as the patient and/or surrogate decision makers have had time to discuss and deliberate about goals and desired outcomes. Ideally, as mentioned above, this will be completed well before it is actually needed for guidance as end of life approaches.

Bradley C. Buckhout, M.D.

Appendix B

The following is a typical POLST document:

HIPAA PERMITS DISCLOSURE OF POLST TO OTHER HEALTH CARE PROVIDERS AS NECESSARY

Physician Orders for Life-Sustaining Treatment (POLST)
First, follow these orders, then contact Physician/NP/PA.
A copy of the signed POLST form is a legally valid physician order. Any section not completed implies full treatment for that section. POLST complements an Advance Directive and is not intended to replace that document.

Patient Last Name: Date Form Prepared:
Patient First Name:
Patient Middle Name:
Patient Date of Birth:
Medical Record #: (optional)

A
CARDIOPULMONARY RESUSCITATION (CPR): If patient has no pulse and is not breathing.
If patient is NOT in cardiopulmonary arrest, follow orders in Sections B and C.
Check One:
o Attempt Resuscitation/CPR (Selecting CPR in Section A requires selecting Full Treatment in Section B)
o Do Not Attempt Resuscitation/DNR (Allow Natural Death)

B

MEDICAL INTERVENTIONS: If patient is found with a pulse and/or is breathing.

Check One:

o Full Treatment – primary goal of prolonging life by all medically effective means. In addition to treatment described in Selective Treatment and Comfort-Focused Treatment, use intubation, advanced airway interventions, mechanical ventilation, and cardioversion as indicated.

o Trial Period of Full Treatment.

o Selective Treatment – goal of treating medical conditions while avoiding burdensome measures. In addition to treatment described in Comfort-Focused Treatment, use medical treatment, IV antibiotics, and IV fluids as indicated. Do not intubate. May use non-invasive positive airway pressure. Generally avoid intensive care.

o Request transfer to hospital only if comfort needs cannot be met in current location.

o Comfort-Focused Treatment – primary goal of maximizing comfort. Relieve pain and suffering with medication by any route as needed; use oxygen, suctioning, and manual treatment of airway obstruction. Do not use treatments listed in Full and Selective Treatment unless consistent with comfort goal. Request transfer to hospital only if comfort needs cannot be met in current location.

Additional Orders:

_____
_____
_____

Bradley C. Buckhout, M.D.

C
ARTIFICIALLY ADMINISTERED NUTRITION: Offer food by mouth if feasible and desired.

Check One:

o Long-term artificial nutrition, including feeding tubes. Additional Orders:

___

o Trial period of artificial nutrition, including feeding tubes.

___

o No artificial means of nutrition, including feeding tubes.

D
INFORMATION AND SIGNATURES:

Check One:

Discussed with:

o Patient (Patient Has Capacity)

o Legally Recognized Decision maker (surrogate)

___

o AdvanceDirective dated:_____ Available and reviewed Health Care Agent if named in Advance Directive:

___

o Advance Directive not available Name:

___

o No Advance Directive

Surrogate Phone: _____

Signature of Physician / Nurse Practitioner / Physician Assistant (Physician/NP/PA)

When Caring Trumps Curing

My signature below indicates to the best of my knowledge that these orders are consistent with the patient's medical condition and preferences.

Print Physician/NP/PA Name:
Physician/NP/PA Phone #:
Physician/PA License #, NP Cert. #:

Physician/NP/PA Signature: (required)
_____

Signature of Patient or Legally Recognized Decision maker
_____
I am aware that this form is voluntary. By signing this form, the legally recognized decision maker acknowledges that this request regarding resuscitative measures is consistent with the known desires of, and with the best interest of, the individual who is the subject of the form.

Print Name:
Relationship: (write self if patient)

Signature: (required)
Date:

- Completing a POLST form is voluntary.
- POLST does not replace the Advance Directive. When available, review the Advance Directive and POLST form to ensure consistency, and update forms appropriately to resolve any conflicts.
- POLST must be completed by a health care provider based on patient preferences and medical indications.

Bradley C. Buckhout, M.D.

- A legally recognized decision maker may include a court-appointed conservator or guardian, agent designated in an Advance Directive, orally designated surrogate, spouse, registered domestic partner, parent of a minor, closest available relative, or person whom the patient's physician/NP/PA believes best knows what is in the patient's best interest and will make decisions in accordance with the patient's expressed wishes and values to the extent known.
- A legally recognized decision maker may execute the POLST form only if the patient lacks capacity or has designated that the decision maker's authority is effective immediately.
- To be valid a POLST form must be signed by (1) a physician, or by a nurse practitioner or a physician assistant acting under the supervision of a physician and within the scope of practice authorized by law and (2) the patient or decision maker. Verbal orders are acceptable with follow-up signature by physician/NP/PA in accordance with facility/community policy.
- If a translated form is used with patient or decision maker, attach it to the signed English POLST form.
- Use of original form is strongly encouraged. Photocopies and FAXes of signed POLST forms are legal and valid. A copy should be retained in patient's medical record, on Ultra Pink paper when possible.

POLST forms are different in each state. The order of the sections or the options within a section may be different but they cover the same information. Below provides information about the forms. If you have any questions, talk to your health care professional.

When Caring Trumps Curing

Section A: Cardiopulmonary Resuscitation (CPR) only applies when the patient is unresponsive, has no pulse and is not breathing.

Check one of the following:
    Attempt Resuscitation / CPR
    Do Not Attempt Resuscitation / DNR
If patient is not in cardiopulmonary arrest go to section B & C
This is similar to a Do-No-Resuscitate Order (DNR Order), but a patient only has a DNR Order when they do not want CPR. The POLST form allows patients to clearly show they DO want CPR. If neither is checked, EMS personel will provide CPR if medically indicated.

Section B: Medical Interventions (patient has pulse and is breathing)

Check one of the following:
    Comfort Measures Only: Provide care to relieve pain and suffering through the use of any medications by any route. Positioning, wound care, etc. Use oxygen, suction, manual treatment for airway obstruction as needed for comfort. Preference No Hospital transfer, unless comfort needs cannot be met here.
    Treatment Plan: Provide treatment through symptom control.
    Limited Treatment: In addition to comfort care, use medical treatments, antibiotics, fluids, cardiac monitoring as needed. No intubation, advanced airway or mechanical ventilation. Non-invasive support (CPAP, BiPAP) OK if necessary. Transfer to hospital if needed, avoid ICU.
    Treatment Plan: Provide Basic medical care.
    Full Treatment: in addition to above use intubation, mechanical ventilation if needed. Hospital transfer including ICU

Bradley C. Buckhout, M.D.

Treatment Plan: all treatment including mechanical ventilation. This section gives medical orders when CPR is not required but the patient still has a medical emergency and cannot communicate. There are three options and a space for a health care professional to write in orders specific for the patient. Care is always provided to patients. This section is just for letting emergency personnel know what treatments the patient wants to have.

In many states, if a patient chooses CPR or leaves Section A blank, he/she is required to choose "Full Treatment" in Section B. This is because CPR usually requires intubation and a breathing machine, which are only options under "Full Treatment".

This section is the heart of the POLST form. If a patient has a medical emergency but does not want CPR this is the section emergency personnel will look at to see whether the patient wants to go to the hospital or not (for Full Treatment and Limited Interventions - yes; for Comfort Measures Only - no). If the patient only has a DNR order, emergency personnel would take them to the hospital.

Section C: Artificially Administered Nutrition

Check one of the following:
- Long term artificial nutrition by feeding tube
- Defined trial period of tube feeding
- No artificial feeding by tube

Additional (define trial period or goals)

This section is where orders are given about artificial nutrition (and in some states artificial hydration) for when the patient cannot eat. All POLST forms state that patients should always be offered food by mouth if possible.

Other Section: Signatures

Healthcare professional: Since this form is a medical order a health care professional is required to sign it in order for it to be valid. Which health care professionals can sign (nurse, doctor) varies by state. The form has a statement saying that, by signing the form, the healthcare professional agrees that the orders on the form match what treatments the patient said he/she wanted during a medical emergency based on his/her medical condition today.

Patient or Surrogate: Most states require the patient or his/her surrogate to sign this form. This helps to show the patient or surrogate was part of the conversation and agrees with the orders listed on the form.

Bradley C. Buckhout, M.D.

Appendix C

Do not regret growing older, it is a privilege denied to many.

If you are depressed, you are living in the past.
If you are anxious, you are living in the future.
If you are at peace, you are living in the present. - Lao Tzu

"I am the master of my fate: I am the captain of my soul."

William Ernest Henley, Echoes of Life and Death

The following is a representative list of resources for those interested in further study and explanation. The resources are much more extensive than this list and these may serve as a starting point for your exploration.

Websites:

Coalition for Compassionate Care of California:
  coalitionccc.org
a multi-disciplinary organization to create a community where people explore their wishes for care towards the end of life, express these wishes, and have their wishes honored.

National Hospice & Palliative Care Organization nhpco.org
provides the history of hospice and palliative care, finding a provider and much more.

When Caring Trumps Curing

My Wish gowish.org this site provides a list of items and a grid on which to place them dependent on the degree of importance for you. A helpful way to consider topics and discuss them with your loved ones.
Examples: "Not being short of breath",
"Having someone who will listen to me."
These can be ranked as: Very Important, Somewhat Important, Not Very Important.

National Healthcare Decisions Day nhdd.org A key goal of NHDD is to demystify healthcare decision-making and make the topic of advance care planning inescapable.
On NHDD (April 16 each year), no one in the U.S. should be able to open a paper, watch TV, view the internet, see a physician or lawyer, or go to a healthcare facility without being presented with the topic of advance care planning. Among other things, NHDD helps people understand that advance health care decision-making includes much more than living wills; it is a process that should focus first on conversation and choosing an agent.

There are literally thousands of other websites to search using advanced care planning or advanced directives as your search topic.

Bradley C. Buckhout, M.D.

Books

Death and Dying by Elizabeth Kuebler-Ross
Being Mortal: Medicine and What Matters in the End
    Atul Gwande M.D.
At Peace by Samuel Harrington
A Better Way of Dying by Jeanne Fitzpatrick M.D. & Eileen
    Fitzpatrick J.D.
Tuesdays with Morrie by Mitch Albom
The Good Death by Marilyn Webb
Long Goodbye by William Colby
I'll Have It My Way by Hattie Bryant
Life after Life by Raymond Moody, M.D., Ph.D.
From Death to Rebirth - Teachings of Pekka Ervast

Notes

1. Ouchi, Kei et al. Prognosis After Emergency Department Intubation to Inform Shared Decision-Making. Journal of American Geriatric Society 2018 15March. https://doi.org/10.1111/jgs.15361
2. Morbidity and Mortality Weekly Report (MMWR) Jan 1, 2016/64(50);1378-82

Bradley C. Buckhout, M.D.

www.ingramcontent.com/pod-product-compliance
Lightning Source LLC
Chambersburg PA
CBHW071426180526
45170CB00001B/236